# THE TRUTH ABOUT ILLNESS AND DISEASE

# THE TRUTH ABOUT ILLNESS AND DISEASE

Robert N. Golden, M.D.
University of Wisconsin–Madison
*General Editor*

Fred L. Peterson, Ph.D.
University of Texas–Austin
*General Editor*

Carla Weiland,
with Karen Weiland,
M.S. R.N., C.N.P., C.D.E.

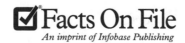

An imprint of Infobase Publishing

Facts On File, Inc.
An imprint of Infobase Publishing
132 West 31st Street
New York, NY 10001

Library of Congress Cataloging-in-Publication Data

The truth about illness and disease / [edited by] Robert N. Golden, Fred L. Peterson.
    p. cm.
  Includes index.
  ISBN-13: 978-0-8160-7635-2 (hardcover : alk. paper)
  ISBN-10: 0-8160-7635-9 (hardcover : alk. paper) 1. Medicine, Popular. I. Golden, Robert N. II. Peterson, Fred. L.
  RC81.T865 2009
  616.003—dc22

                                                    2009000597

Facts On File books are available at special discounts when purchased in bulk quantities for businesses, associations, institutions or sales promotions. Please call our Special Sales Department in New York at (212) 967-8800 or (800) 322-8755.

You can find Facts On File on the World Wide Web at http://www.factsonfile.com

Text design by David Strelecky

Printed and bound in United States of America

MP MSRF 10 9 8 7 6 5 4 3 2 1

This book is printed on acid-free paper.

# CONTENTS

# LIST OF ILLUSTRATIONS

# PREFACE

The Truth About series—updated and expanded to include 20 volumes—seeks to identify the most pressing health issues and social challenges confronting our nation's youth. Adolescence is the period between the onset of puberty and the attainment of adulthood. Adolescence is also a time of storm, stress, and risk-taking for many young people. During adolescence, a person's health is influenced by biological, psychological, and social factors, all of which interact with one's environment—family, peers, school, and community. It is a time when teenagers experience profound changes.

With the latest available statistics and new insights that have emerged from ongoing research, the Truth About series seeks to help young people build a foundation of information as they face some of the challenges that will affect their health and well-being. These challenges include high-risk behaviors, such as drinking, smoking, and other drug use; sexual behaviors that can lead to adolescent pregnancy and sexually transmitted diseases (STDs), such as HIV/AIDS; mental-health concerns, such as depression and suicide; learning disorders and disabilities, which are often associated with school failures and school dropouts; serious family problems, including domestic violence and abuse; and lifestyle factors, which increase adolescents' risk for noncommunicable diseases, such as diabetes and cardiovascular disease, among others.

Broader underlying factors also influence adolescent health. These include socioeconomic circumstances, such as poverty, available health care, and the political and social situations in which young people live. Although these factors can negatively affect adolescent health and well-being, as well as school performance, many of these negative health outcomes are preventable with the proper knowledge and information.

With prevention in mind, the writers and editors of each topical volume in the Truth About series have tried to provide cutting-edge information that is supported by research and scientific evidence. Vital facts are presented that inform youth about the challenges experienced during adolescence, while special features seek to dispel common myths and misconceptions. Some of the main topics explored include abuse, alcohol, death and dying, divorce, drugs, eating disorders, family life, fear and depression, rape, sexual behavior and unplanned pregnancy, smoking, and violence. All volumes discuss risk-taking behaviors and their consequences, healthy choices, prevention, available treatments, and where to get help.

In this new edition of the series, we also have added eight new titles in areas of increasing significance to today's youth. ADHD, or attention-deficit/hyperactivity disorder, and learning disorders are diagnosed with increasing frequency, and many students have observed or know of classmates receiving treatment for these conditions, even if they have not themselves received this diagnosis. Gambling is gaining currency in our culture, as casinos open and expand in many parts of the country, and the Internet offers easy access for this addictive behavior. Another consequence of our increasingly "online" society, unfortunately, is the presence of online predators. Environmental hazards represent yet another danger, and it is important to provide unbiased information about this topic to our youth. Suicide, which for many years has been a "silent epidemic," is now gaining recognition as a major public health problem throughout the life span, including the teenage and young adult years. We now also offer an overview of illness and disease in a volume that includes the major conditions of particular interest and concern to youth. In addition to illness, however, it is essential to emphasize health and its promotion, and this is especially apparent in the volumes on physical fitness and stress management.

It is our intent that each book serve as an accessible, authoritative resource that young people can turn to for accurate and meaningful answers to their specific questions. The series can help them research particular problems and provide an up-to-date evidence base. It is also designed with parents, teachers, and counselors in mind so that they have a reliable resource that they can share with youth who seek their guidance.

Finally, we have tried to provide unbiased facts rather than subjective opinions. Our goal is to help elevate the health of the public with an emphasis on its most precious component—our youth. As young people face the challenges of an increasingly complex world, we as educators want them to be armed with the most powerful weapon available—knowledge.

Robert N. Golden, M.D.
Fred L. Peterson, Ph.D.
General Editors

# HOW TO USE THIS BOOK

## NOTE TO STUDENTS

Knowledge is power. By possessing knowledge you have the ability to make decisions, ask follow-up questions, and know where to go to obtain more information. In the world of health, that is power! That is the purpose of this book—to provide you the power you need to obtain unbiased, accurate information and *The Truth About Illness and Disease.*

Topics in each volume of The Truth About are arranged in alphabetical order, from A to Z. Each of these entries defines its topic and explains in detail the particular issue. At the end of most entries are cross-references to related topics. A list of all topics by letter can be found in the table of contents or at the back of the book in the index.

How have these books been compiled? First, the publisher worked with me to identify some of the country's leading authorities on key issues in health education. These individuals were asked to identify some of the major concerns that young people have about such topics. The writers read the literature, spoke with health experts, and incorporated their own life and professional experiences to pull together the most up-to-date information on health issues, particularly those of interest to adolescents and of concern in Healthy People 2010.

Throughout the alphabetical entries, the reader will find sidebars that separate Fact from Fiction. There are Question-and-Answer boxes that attempt to address the most common questions that youth ask about sensitive topics. In addition, readers will find a special feature called "Teens Speak"—case studies of teens with personal stories related to the topic in hand.

This may be one of the most important books you will ever read. Please share it with your friends, families, teachers, and classmates. Remember, you possess the power to control your future. One way to affect your course is through the acquisition of knowledge. Good luck and keep healthy.

## NOTE TO LIBRARIANS

This book, along with the rest of the series The Truth About, serves as a wonderful resource for young researchers. It contains a variety of facts, case studies, and further readings that the reader can use to help answer questions, formulate new questions, or determine where to go to find more information. Even though the topics may be considered delicate by some, don't be afraid to ask patrons if they have questions. Feel free to direct them to the appropriate sources, but do not press them if you encounter reluctance. The best we can do as educators is to let young people know that we are there when they need us.

Robert N. Golden, M.D.
Fred L. Peterson, Ph.D.
General Editors

# FIGHTING ILLNESS AND DISEASE

The word *disease* has different meanings for different people. For someone who is young, relatively healthy, and living in North America, disease might seem like something that happens to older people or something that happens mostly in other countries. In some respects, that is true. The older one gets the more susceptible to disease a person becomes, due to two factors.

First, as people age, their **genes** age and become more susceptible to defects that may have been encoded at conception. Another factor is that any unhealthy personal habits such as smoking have had more time to affect the body and its cells. For instance, a 55-year-old male may have a 30-year smoking habit that has caused his cells to change during replication. This unhealthy habit may have set him up for cancer or other diseases.

Certainly, someone growing up in America is not as susceptible to some diseases, such as malaria and measles, as people in some other countries. For some people in Africa and Asia, for example, the potential of mosquito bites to cause malaria and change one's health is a serious threat.

Another factor contributing to the spread of disease in many countries is the difficulty of locating a safe supply of drinking water. It is not uncommon for children in many countries to develop severe diarrhea and die of **dehydration.** Dying from a lack of water is not something most people think of happening in America. Yet, according to a government study called *Global Trends 2015,* access to safe drinking water in the United States will worsen by 2015. Many ecologic or "green" efforts try to address the issue of safe drinking water, particularly runoff from fertilizers and some farms.

1

Increasingly, Americans—even young Americans—battle disease every day. With 66 percent of Americans overweight, and 51 percent of American children overweight, diabetes experts warn us of the secondary effects of obesity that the younger generation will experience. Due to the unprecedented early development of Type 2 diabetes in youth, some experts are even predicting a lowering of life expectancy for the younger generation—for the first time in the nation's history. There are many factors contributing to this anticipated trend of less healthy people, but two of them are easy to identify: ready access to high-fat, high-calorie foods, and less physical activity. Furthermore, complications of Type 2 diabetes are serious: **cardiovascular disease**, high **cholesterol**, and hypertension—diseases and conditions for which teens and young adults will be increasingly at risk. The nation is beginning to see the need for adolescents to have medications and surgery to correct these diseases.

## TYPES OF DISEASES AND ILLNESSES

**Infectious** diseases, or those caused by **viruses**, **bacteria**, **parasites**, and other living organisms, are everywhere. Although the **vaccines** and **antibiotics** used to control them once brought hope that they would be eradicated, infectious diseases are still a major cause of death in the developing world. In fact, there is an international resurgence of some diseases. In addition, a serious threat of infection comes from the bacteria that live normally in the human body. These pose a serious threat of infection when the body's resistance is lowered. Bacteria can multiply rapidly—one bacterium in the body can replicate into 16,777,220 bacteria within a day. If the bacteria are resistant to antibiotics and spread to other people, an epidemic can result. The overuse of antibiotics in some regions, including the United States, has resulted in bacteria mutating to more powerful and less treatable pathogens. Either new antibiotics must be discovered continually to treat the mutated bacteria or the disease will not be effectively treated.

**Chronic** diseases, or illnesses that last a long period of time, are usually not completely cured. Cancer, diabetes, heart disease, Alzheimer's disease, and AIDS are examples of chronic diseases. In 2005, more than 133 million Americans had chronic illnesses, and more than 75 percent of the money spent on medical care in the United States in that year was spent on treating chronic diseases. Although research continues in search of cures for chronic diseases, scientists have not yet developed cures for diseases such as diabetes or Alzheimer's.

Because the cures are difficult, more and more research is aimed at discovering how to prevent these diseases in the first place. As the American health-care system has historically focused on treatment rather than prevention, the shift to a focus on prevention has proved difficult.

## MENTAL DISORDERS

Mental disorders are another type of illness. These include developmental, emotional, and behavioral problems. At least one in five youths suffers from such an illness. One of the major health problems facing the United States is preventing and treating such diseases.

During adolescence, the brains of teenagers undergo significant changes, as do their emotions, **hormones,** behavior, and interpersonal relationships. Many chronic mental disorders can start during adolescence and then carry over into adulthood. The range of health behaviors acquired in the teen years that influence adult medical health include the use of substances and dietary and exercise habits. These in turn can determine the development of cardiovascular disease, diabetes, obesity, osteoporosis, and HIV/AIDS. In recent years, research has confirmed that mental disorders are relatively common in adolescence. For example, 20 to 30 percent of adolescents report symptoms of **depression;** more than half of young people have used an illicit drug by the time of their high school graduation; and from 9 to 21 percent of adolescents have **anxiety** disorders in a 12-month period.

### Mood Disorders

One type of mental illness is mood disorders, which includes depression and **bipolar disorder.** Fifty years ago, the age of onset for depression was 30; now it is about 15. When it occurs, it often has a great impact on school performance and interpersonal relationships.

Depression is characterized by intense feelings of sadness, hopelessness, worthlessness, and listlessness. Bipolar disorder does not occur as often as depression; it too has an onset during adolescence. Bipolar disorder is characterized by a distinct period of abnormally and persistently elevated or irritable mood lasting for at least one week, with three or more of the following symptoms also occurring: inflated self-esteem, decreased need for sleep, talkativeness, flight of ideas, distractibility, and involvement in risk-taking, pleasurable activities have run a high potential for painful consequences.

Suicide is now the third leading cause of death in adolescents. It is more common in males than females, but females have more reported attempts at suicide. Recognition of symptoms that go beyond typical teenage mood changes is one of the challenges in the prevention of suicide. Another is that, while antidepressants have improved significantly for adult use, they do not always work the same way in adolescents, and some patients complain of worsened symptoms.

### Anxiety Disorders

Another type of mental illness is anxiety disorder, which includes **generalized anxiety disorder,** panic disorder, obsessive-compulsive disorder, **post-traumatic stress disorder,** phobias, separation anxiety disorder, and social anxiety disorder. Although the incidence of each of these is low in teens, taken together, these disorders are relatively common. Separation anxiety disorder and phobias are more common in early childhood than in adolescence. There is increased incidence of panic disorder and agoraphobia during adolescence. While most fears and shyness are normal during the teen years, anxiety disorders are different. They interfere with regular functioning in a person's life in school, friendships, family, and work. Symptoms of generalized anxiety disorder are persistent worrying the person cannot seem to shake, fatigue, muscle tension, muscle aches, difficulty swallowing, trembling, twitching, irritability, sweating, and hot flashes.

### Eating Disorders

**Anorexia nervosa** (self-imposed starvation) and **bulimia** (overeating and then purging) are the two major eating disorders. Typically, these disorders start in the early teen years, when young people are most susceptible due to the increase in the daily energy requirements needed to support normal growth and development. Girls have a 50 percent increase in caloric requirements, and boys have an 80 percent increase.

Dieting is also common among teens who want to change their images. Two of every three female high school students are trying to lose weight. Treatment of anorexia nervosa is most effective when initiated early, and, for long-term success, effective treatment requires focus on psychological and self-esteem issues rather than just on weight gain. About half of those diagnosed with anorexia nervosa will make a full recovery. Approximately 6 percent will die from complications of the disease.

## CAUSES OF DISEASE AND ILLNESS

Bacteria, protists, and viruses are the pathogens that cause infectious diseases, which spread from person to person by direct or indirect contact. Some pathogens are transferred through the air or through contaminated food and water. When people who have colds or measles sneeze, cough, or even talk and laugh, they send sprays of tiny water droplets of mucus into the air. If the droplets contain **pathogens** and are breathed in by another person, that person may become sick. Some pathogens, such as those that cause the flu, whooping cough, or tuberculosis (TB), can survive even when the infected droplets dry out and float like dust particles.

Vectors, animals that are able to transmit diseases to humans, include mosquitoes, ticks and other bugs, flies, rats, bats, and dogs. Female mosquitoes, the most harmful vectors, spread malaria as well as other diseases by penetrating the skin and feeding on blood while they inject the pathogens found in their saliva. Ticks spread Lyme disease, and dogs, bats, and other mammals spread rabies.

Changes and defects in genes, the basic hereditary units that determine one's characteristics, can cause diseases when the faulty gene is passed from parent to child. Some of the diseases are present at birth, while others occur later in life. Cystic fibrosis is an example of a disease in which a single gene has mutated or changed. **Down syndrome** is an example of a disease in which the genes on a chromosome are arranged abnormally. Diabetes and **congenital** heart disease are examples in which the interaction of genes and the environment contribute to the disease.

Scientists predict that if the global temperature continues to rise as it has (1 degree Fahrenheit in the last 100 years), everyone will experience an increase in health problems. According to a U.S. Department of Agriculture report, over the last 40 to 50 years, the amount of ragweed pollen has doubled due to the increase in carbon dioxide, the main food source for plant growth. The number of people who suffer hay fever, an allergic reaction to pollen, is expected to rise above the current rate of one in every five Americans.

More potential allergy and asthma triggers, ozone and smog, are expected to increase with warmer temperatures. A warmer climate will support disease-carrying mosquitoes in places that previously were too cold for them to survive. In the Andes Mountains of Columbia, for example, mosquitoes that were never found above 3,300 feet have recently been found at 7,200 feet.

With the onset of globalization, record numbers of people are traveling all over the world. The rapid movement of people over long distances means that a disease can spread with extraordinary speed. Air travelers can introduce diseases to areas of the world that have never experienced them before, meaning that people will have no resistance to them.

Mental illnesses can also "spread" or increase in occurrences. One contributor to some mental disorders is social pressure, which is also magnified by the media. Bombarded by images of "perfect" bodies, people can become obsessed with self-image, sometimes to the point of having lowered self-esteem. Feeling bad about oneself can lead to eating disorders, anxieties, and **addictions.**

## PREVENTION

Young people make decisions every day—which classes to take, what sports to play, what foods to eat, which friends to spend time with, and whether or not to avoid risky or dangerous behaviors. According to the Centers for Disease Control and Prevention (CDC), with more information teens today are making smart decisions about their choices and avoiding risky behavior more than ever before. Teens who make healthy choices are less likely to use alcohol, cigarettes, and drugs, and more likely to achieve their goals.

### Making Healthy Choices

It is one thing to know what safe health behaviors are; it is another to follow through and make good decisions and act in a healthy way.

Good decision-making involves many factors. Being proactive helps by considering what you believe and value before you are put into a situation that could change your life. In the moment with social pressure around, one might make a very different decision. Getting good information and knowing your choices about your physical and mental health is important; use reliable Web sites to find good resources in your community. Sometimes you may have to weigh many pros and cons to come to the best decision for you.

There are several healthy ways to promote good decision-making. Learn about balancing your life; learn to deal with the pressures of society, school, and family in healthy ways, such as making time for relaxation or exercise. Work at building your self-confidence and figure out what your values and beliefs are. Over time you will want to learn to stand up for your beliefs in a way that makes you feel comfortable, but this takes practice, like every other skill. Activities such as listing your positive qualities and writing down 10 ways in which you are special may be good ways to get started.

Get vigorous exercise lasting at least 20 minutes a minimum of three times a week and regular exercise daily. Research shows that

## DID YOU KNOW?

# U.S. Youth Risk Behaviors, 1997–2007

|  | 1999 | 2001 | 2003 | 2005 | 2007 |
|---|---|---|---|---|---|
| TOBACCO USE | | | | | |
| Frequent cigarette use | 16.8 | 13.8 | 9.7 | 9.4 | 8.1 |
| ALCOHOL and OTHER DRUG USE | | | | | |
| Episodic heavy drinking | 31.5 | 29.9 | 28.3 | 25.5 | 26.0 |
| Had a least 1 drink on 1 or more days in the last 30 days | 50.0 | 47.1 | 44.9 | 43.3 | 44.7 |
| Lifetime marijuana use | 47.2 | 42.4 | 40.2 | 38.4 | 38.1 |
| Current cocaine use | 4.0 | 4.2 | 4.1 | 3.4 | 3.3 |
| Lifetime illegal steroid use | 3.7 | 5.0 | 6.1 | 4.0 | 3.9 |
| SEXUAL BEHAVIORS | | | | | |
| Used birth control pill before last sexual intercourse | 16.2 | 18.2 | 17.0 | 17.6 | 16.0 |
| Had intercourse with four or more people in lifetime | 16.2 | 14.2 | 14.4 | 14.3 | 14.9 |
| PHYSICAL ACTIVITY | | | | | |
| Attended physical education class daily | 29.1 | 32.2 | 28.4 | 33.0 | 30.3 |

Data are percentages of U.S. high school students.

Source: Youth Risk Behavior Surveillance System, Centers for Disease Control and Prevention, 2007.

exercise is very effective in regulating stress and mood, which can help you make better decisions. This will provide you with an effective lifelong behavior to deal with stress issues. Additionally, eating a nutritious diet with fruits, vegetables, and whole grains while reducing sugary and fried foods adds to the physical balance your body requires.

If you have or suspect you have a health problem—a disease or a disorder—see a health-care provider to get early treatment in order to achieve the best results.

## Avoiding Risky Behaviors

Scientists have discovered through their research of many years that the following seven behaviors should be avoided because they put your health at risk. First, it is unhealthy to eat too much or too little, so you should watch what you eat. Eat safe foods (some foods must be heated to kill bacteria and some must be refrigerated to avoid spoiling).

The second risky behavior is lack of exercise. The lack of exercise is a well-documented reason for increased risk of obesity, diabetes, heart disease, and osteoarthritis.

The third problem is the lack of vaccinations. Vaccines can protect you from infectious diseases that formerly killed huge numbers of people in epidemics.

Another behavior to avoid is smoking. Smoking regularly as a teen makes it likely you will smoke throughout adulthood and put you at high risk for lung cancer, bronchitis, emphysema, and the effects of cardiovascular disease, such as heart attacks or strokes.

The fifth behavior to avoid is stress-related activity. Stress that is not balanced by relaxation can lead to indigestion, headaches, backaches, irritability, anger, and anxiety.

The next behavior to avoid is alcohol and drug abuse. Alcohol and illegal drug use can lead to lifelong problems with substance abuse and can increase the risk of having unsafe, unprotected sex.

The last behavior to avoid is risky sexual behavior. Unsafe sexual practices can result in STDs, HIV infection and AIDS, and unintended pregnancy.

This book covers the diseases and health issues that can affect everyone, young and old. It also provides valuable information about the causes and treatments of these conditions. Perhaps most important to you will be the sections on prevention. It is in fact easier to prevent most diseases than it is to treat them.

## RISKY BUSINESS SELF-TEST

The following self-test is designed to let you find out more about your own risk of catching an infectious disease or contracting a chronic one. To identify whether or not you may be at risk, record your answers to this short true-or-false test on a sheet of paper.

A. Are you at risk of catching an infectious disease?

> 1. I am overdue for recommended vaccinations such as tetanus, polio, and chicken pox.

2. I have had unprotected sex.

3. I have had sex with more than one person.

4. In the past 12 months I have gotten a tattoo or body piercing.

5. I sometimes eat raw or undercooked eggs or meat or drink unpasteurized fruit drinks or milk.

6. When I am close to someone with a cold, flu, or other infectious disease, I don't take special measures to avoid catching it.

7. When I go into an area where there might be ticks, I don't take any special precautions.

B. Are you at risk of getting a chronic disease?

1. I only protect my skin from the Sun if I expect to be outdoors a long time.

2. In the past 30 days, I have had a beer, glass of wine, or other type of alcohol more than four times.

3. In the past 30 days, I have been drunk four times.

4. I am highly stressed most of the time.

5. I smoke cigarettes.

6. I live in a household with a cigarette smoker.

7. I have occasionally ridden in a car with a driver who has been drinking.

8. I am overweight.

9. I am preoccupied much of the time with thinking about food and my weight.

10. I eat about two servings of fruits and vegetables every day.

11. I do at least 20 minutes of vigorous physical activity twice a week.

## Scoring
### Part A
Answering "true" to any of these seven questions means that you are at risk for contracting an infectious disease. Without appropriate vaccinations, you are at risk of getting several "childhood" diseases. If

you get vaccinated against diseases, you will never get them. **Hepatitis B,** usually transmitted through sexual activity, is preventable by the hepatitis B vaccine. Having unprotected sex puts you at risk of getting a sexually transmitted disease (STD). The best way for those who are sexually active to reduce the risk of getting an STD is to always use a latex condom. Having a mutually monogamous relationship also reduces the risk. The more partners a person has, the greater the chances of getting an STD.

Using unsterilized needles and piercing tools for body piercings and tattoos can carry infectious agents for hepatitis B and C and HIV. Infectious agents can spread in materials such as water and foods such as undercooked poultry and spoiled milk.

Taking precautions against colds and influenza (flu) will reduce these viral diseases that spread via airborne droplets, such as those in a cough or sneeze. People with these diseases usually have germs on their hands as well, so touching something they touch can spread the disease. If you spend time in tall grass or woodlands you should wear long sleeves and long pants and check often for ticks. Otherwise you are increasing your risk of getting Lyme disease, which is transmitted to humans through deer ticks.

## Part B
Answering "true" to any of these 11 statements means you are making some choices that put you at risk for developing a chronic disease. You are putting yourself at high risk for developing skin cancer if you often expose your skin to sunlight. The longer and more frequent the exposure, the higher the risk. By excessive drinking, you put yourself at greater risk for chronic diseases such as heart disease, cancer, and **cirrhosis** of the liver. Choosing to drink alcohol immediately puts a teenager at greater risk of homicide, suicide, or a motor vehicle accident. Drinking can affect school and sports performance. Teens that are drinking are at risk to have unsafe sex and to get in legal trouble.

You may be at risk for stress-related illnesses including asthma, headaches, and various skin problems. If you smoke, the odds of your getting a **respiratory** illness (like bronchitis) are higher than normal. The American Cancer Society cites cigarette smoking as responsible for more than 30 percent of cancer deaths and as a major cause of heart disease.

By riding with someone who has been drinking, you are risking your life and those of all your passengers. More than 20 percent of teens' auto deaths are alcohol-related.

Obesity puts you at greater risk for heart disease, high blood pressure, diabetes, cancer, and stroke. Whether it is the result of poor nutrition, lack of exercise, or binge eating, being seriously overweight raises the risk of depression, coronary heart disease, diabetes, and stroke.

If you have low self-esteem, you are at risk of being or becoming anorexic or bulimic. Eating less than five servings of fruits and vegetables a day puts you at risk for both cancer and heart disease. People who eat five servings of fruit and vegetables a day were half as likely to develop cancer of the digestive and respiratory tract as those who ate fewer servings a day. Without adequate exercise, you are increasing your risk of getting cardiovascular diseases. In the short term, too little exercise can affect people's energy levels, mood, and stamina. Over the long term, inactivity raises the risk of heart disease and being overweight, which puts you at risk for many other diseases.

# A TO Z ENTRIES

# ■ ADHD (ATTENTION DEFICIT/HYPERACTIVITY DISORDER)

A condition in which it is hard to control behavior and pay attention. Inattention, **hyperactivity,** and impulsivity are the main symptoms of ADHD. Because most children have some level of these characteristics at least some time in their lives, it is important that a qualified health-care provider thoroughly examine and diagnose a child who might have the condition. Often this might be a pediatrician or pediatric professional specializing in ADHD diagnosis and treatment.

## SYMPTOMS

Symptoms of impulsiveness and hyperactivity may appear a year or more before symptoms of inattentiveness begin. Although children's self-control may vary with their different environments, ADHD may be suspected due to hyperactivity, distractibility, and poor concentration affecting performance in school, as well as family and social relationships.

### Hyperactivity

Hyperactive children seem to be constantly in motion, playing with whatever is in sight or talking nonstop. Sitting still is a difficult task for them. Hyperactive teens and adults may need to stay busy and do several things at once, and they feel restless inside.

### Impulsivity

Impulsive children have difficulty thinking before they act and follow their immediate reactions without thinking about the consequences. As teens and adults, they may do things that provide small, immediate gratification, rather than deciding on and following through with things that have greater long-term benefits.

### Inattentiveness

Signs of inattention include becoming distracted easily, failing to pay attention to details, and skipping from one activity to another.

## DIAGNOSIS

A diagnosis of ADHD requires that the symptomatic behaviors be shown to the degree appropriate for the person's age. (Children at younger ages display the symptoms at a lesser level than older children.) The symptoms must appear before age seven and continue for at least six months, and they must create a real handicap in at least two areas of a person's life such as in school, on the playground, at home, or in the community. So someone could show some symptoms, but if his or her schoolwork or friendships are not impaired by these behaviors, the person would not be diagnosed with ADHD. To assess whether a child has ADHD, specialists consider several important questions: Are the behaviors excessive, ongoing, and pervasive? That is, do they occur more often than in other children of the same age? Are they a continuous problem? Do the behaviors occur in several situations?

Often apparent in preschool and early school-age children, ADHD affects between 3 and 5 percent of children in the United States; that's approximately 2 million children. Parents and guardians, guidance counselors, and school personnel can provide help and support for children with ADHD to achieve their full potential.

## CAUSES

Most research shows that ADHD arises from biological causes and not from the home environment. Environmental factors may influence the severity of the disorder but do not seem to give rise to the disorder itself. According to the National Institute of Mental Health, studies have shown a possible correlation between ADHD in a child and the use of cigarettes and alcohol by the mother during pregnancy. Other studies show that 25 percent of the close relatives in the families of ADHD children also have ADHD—the rate is about 5 percent in the general population. In addition, many studies of twins now show that there is a strong genetic influence in the disorder. Researchers are trying to identify the **genes** that place a person at risk to develop ADHD.

## DISORDERS ASSOCIATED WITH ADHD

About 20 to 30 percent of children with ADHD also have a specific learning disability. The disabilities can include difficulty in understanding certain sounds or words, difficulty with self-expression, reading or spelling disabilities, and writing and arithmetic difficulties.

### Conduct Disorder

About 20 to 40 percent of children with ADHD may eventually develop conduct disorder, which is a pattern of antisocial behavior. Conduct disorder may include lying, stealing, fighting, bullying, destroying property, and carrying or using weapons.

## Oppositional Defiant Disorder

One-third to one-half of children with ADHD—mostly boys—have oppositional defiant disorder. Children with this disorder are temperamental, belligerent, defiant, and argumentative.

## Tourette's Syndrome

Very few children have Tourette's syndrome, a neurological disorder resulting in nervous tics and repetitive mannerisms, such as eye blinks, facial twitches, or grimacing. Many of those children with Tourette's syndrome have ADHD as well. Medications may be used to treat both disorders.

## Anxiety and Depression

Anxiety and depression can occur along with ADHD; treatment of the anxiety or depression can help children with problems of ADHD, and conversely, improving ADHD symptoms can positively impact a child's anxiety if the child can concentrate better and successfully complete tasks.

## COPING AND TREATMENT

ADHD treatment can include medication and/or behavioral therapy, emotional counseling, and practical support. No single treatment works for all children.

Stimulants are the medications most prescribed for ADHD. For adults, a stimulant will generally increase wakefulness. These drugs have been around for many years—one of their uses was to keep adults awake and functioning during war. But they can be addictive for adults and are rarely prescribed for adults anymore. They may make an adult anxious and cause weight loss. Thus, it would seem wrong to give a stimulant to an ADHD child. However, these drugs increase serotonin, a neurotransmitter in the brain that has calming effects, and have been found to be effective for children in lower doses. Basically these drugs allow the brain to inhibit itself, allowing the child to focus on the right thing at the right time, be less distracted, and be less impulsive. This allows the child to function in school, perform other activities better, and be more successful.

There are no known natural treatments for ADHD that have been proven effective scientifically, although a search of the Internet will show many entities pushing for special diets or supplements instead of stimulants. However, 75 percent of ADHD sufferers who go on stimulants gain a benefit from these drugs. One side effect that is watched carefully is weight loss or lack of weight gain in children. Weight gain is an important part of growth, and stimulants may make it difficult for some children to gain or to lose weight.

Another drug, Strattera, also can treat ADHD. It is a nonstimulant medication that works similarly to **antidepressants** by inhibiting the body's uptake of the neurotransmitter **norepinephrine.** This creates a calming effect. The stimulants primarily work on the neurotransmitter **dopamine.** Both of these neurotransmitters are believed to play a role in ADHD.

Though a child's schoolwork and behavior can improve soon after starting medication, the medication does not cure ADHD. It controls the symptoms on the day it is taken. Medication can help the child concentrate better and complete schoolwork, but the drugs do not increase knowledge or improve academic skills. About 80 percent of children who need medication for ADHD still need it as teenagers. More than 50 percent need medication as adults. Adults often start with a stimulant medication, with antidepressants as the second choice for medication.

### Simple Behavioral Interventions
Children with ADHD may need help in organizing. One simple way parents can help is to establish regimens. Parents should schedule

---

**DID YOU KNOW?**

## Health-Care Providers for ADHD

| Specialty | Can Diagnose ADHD | Can Prescribe Medication, if Needed | Provides Counseling or Training |
|---|---|---|---|
| Psychiatrists | Yes | Yes | Yes |
| Psychologists | Yes | No | Yes |
| Pediatricians or Family Physicians | Yes | Yes | No |
| Neurologists | Yes | Yes | No |
| Clinical Social Workers | Yes | No | Yes |

Different qualifications and services are provided by specialists certified to diagnose ADHD.

Source: National Institute of Mental Health, 1996.

daily activities and, as much as possible, should follow the schedule from waking to bedtime each day. These children need their everyday items to be organized—to have a place for everything and everything in its place. Parents can encourage the use of homework and note-book organizers and stress the importance to the child and teacher of writing down the assignments and bringing home the needed books. They should establish consistent rules and be sure to reward the child who is following the rules and behaving well. These children are used to criticism and have come to expect it, so they need to hear praise.

### Teens and Adults Coping with ADHD

All teens, including those with ADHD, face problems with peer pres-sure, fear of failure in school and social situations, and self-esteem. If you have ADHD, you, like all teens, will be learning to make good deci-sions about alcohol, drugs, and sexual activity. Now more than ever, straightforward rules that you and your parents or guardian can agree upon will help guide you as you become more independent and try new things. Research shows that between 30 and 70 percent of children with ADHD continue to have symptoms in their adult years. With treatment that could include medication, education, and **psychotherapy**, teens and adults with ADHD can bring organization out of the complexities of their lives and channel their energy into positive directions.

*See also:* Anxiety and Mood Disorders

### FURTHER READING

Petersen, Christine. *Does Everyone Have ADHD? A Teen's Guide to Diagnosis and Treatment.* New York: Franklin Watts, 2006.

# ■ AIDS (ACQUIRED IMMUNODEFICIENCY SYNDROME)

A disease caused by a **virus** that attacks the **immune** system, making the infected person susceptible to other diseases. The virus that causes AIDS is called the human immunodeficiency virus, or HIV. Although there is no known cure for AIDS, newer medications are allowing people with AIDS to survive much longer than in the past. Many patients with HIV who have not progressed to AIDS are essentially living with a chronic illness now.

HIV attacks the human immune system directly and destroys the cells whose job it is to identify **pathogens** and distinguish one kind

### DID YOU KNOW?

## AIDS Statistics in the United States

| | |
|---|---|
| 500,000 | Total AIDS deaths, 1981–2006 |
| 56,300 | New cases per year |
| 30 | Minutes before the next person between the ages of 13 and 24 contracts HIV |

Although there have been huge numbers of AIDS deaths in the United States, the disease has caused more than 22 million deaths worldwide.

Source: Centers for Disease Control and Prevention, 2008.

of disease-causing organism from another. Once HIV enters these cells, it reproduces inside them and sends new viruses to infect other cells. Eventually the number of these immune system cells decreases, making the person less able to fight disease. The early phase of HIV infection, while viruses are replicating, lasts six to 12 weeks. In the first eight to 10 weeks, the infected person often suffers night sweats and fever. The person may show few symptoms after this for as long as 10 years but can pass the infection to others through sexual intercourse or blood products.

A person can have HIV without having AIDS. When the number of immune cells left drops to a low enough number, the person is usually diagnosed with AIDS. Prior to that, the person may be HIV-positive in one of the stages of the disease, but does not have the diagnosis of AIDS.

Without a functioning immune system, people with AIDS get diseases, such as tuberculosis or particular skin and pneumonia infections, not normally found in people with healthy immune systems. Although many people with AIDS can survive multiple attacks of such diseases, without antiviral drug therapy, their immune systems usually fail. After about 10 years of HIV infection, they die from a secondary infection from another pathogen.

### HOW HIV IS SPREAD

Like all viruses, HIV can only reproduce inside cells. However, HIV can survive for a short time outside the body in body fluids, such as blood and the fluids produced by the male and female reproductive systems.

HIV can spread from one person to another only if body fluids, including blood, saliva, tears, and semen, from an infected person come in contact with those of an uninfected person. Sexual intercourse is one way this can happen. HIV may also pass from an infected woman to her baby during pregnancy or childbirth or through breast milk. Also, infected blood can spread HIV. Blood transfusions before 1985 sometimes transmitted HIV. (Since 1985, all donated blood in the United States has been tested for HIV before being used in transfusions.) In addition, HIV can spread if an infected drug user shares a needle.

HIV does not live on skin, so it is not spread by such contact with an infected person as hugging, shaking hands, bumping into them while playing sports, or using the same drinking glass.

# Fact Or Fiction?

*You can catch HIV, the virus causing AIDS, by sitting on a toilet seat after someone with AIDS has sat on it.*

**The Facts:** Scientific research shows that HIV is not spread by touching something that a person infected with the virus has touched. HIV is NOT

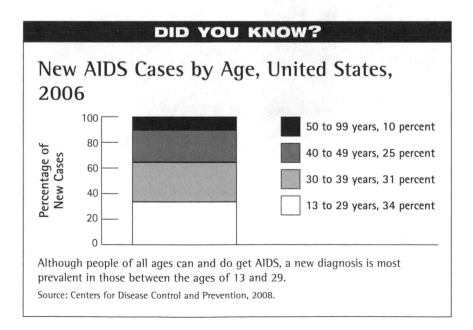

## DID YOU KNOW?

### New AIDS Cases by Age, United States, 2006

Percentage of New Cases

- 50 to 99 years, 10 percent
- 40 to 49 years, 25 percent
- 30 to 39 years, 31 percent
- 13 to 29 years, 34 percent

Although people of all ages can and do get AIDS, a new diagnosis is most prevalent in those between the ages of 13 and 29.

Source: Centers for Disease Control and Prevention, 2008.

transmitted through the air, water, insect bites, or by casual contact such as shaking hands. HIV is transmitted through the exchange of body fluids.

## AIDS AND AGE GROUPS

Information compiled by the Centers for Disease Control and Prevention, the National Center for HIV/AIDS, Viral Hepatitis, STD, and TB Prevention, and the U.S. Department of Health and Human Services, shows that, although new diagnoses are most prevalent in young people ages 13–29, all age groups can be affected by AIDS. The following statistics reflect the number of AIDS cases in the United States between 2001 and 2005:

- 9,101 AIDS cases in children under 13
- 181,802 AIDS cases in females 13 years and older
- 761,723 AIDS cases in males 13 years and older.

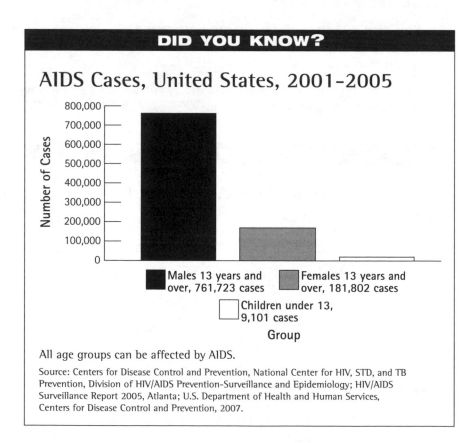

**DID YOU KNOW?**

## AIDS Cases, United States, 2001–2005

All age groups can be affected by AIDS.

Source: Centers for Disease Control and Prevention, National Center for HIV, STD, and TB Prevention, Division of HIV/AIDS Prevention-Surveillance and Epidemiology; HIV/AIDS Surveillance Report 2005, Atlanta; U.S. Department of Health and Human Services, Centers for Disease Control and Prevention, 2007.

## PREVENTIVE BEHAVIORS

There is no cure for AIDS and no **vaccine** to prevent HIV. You can protect yourself from infection by educating yourself about the disease and avoiding any behavior that would allow HIV-infected fluids—blood, semen, vaginal secretions, and breast milk—into your body.

According to the Mayo Clinic, there are additional important ways to prevent HIV infection:

Know the HIV status of any sexual partner and do not engage in unprotected sex unless you are certain your partner is not HIV infected.

Using a new latex (or polyurethane if you are allergic to latex) condom every time you have sex. Lambskin condoms do not protect against HIV. Although condoms can reduce your risk of contracting HIV, they do not eliminate the risk, as condoms can break or develop tears and may not be used properly.

Use only clean, sterile needles to inject drugs; never share needles.

Be aware of risks: Although the number of AIDS deaths in the United States has decreased due to powerful new antiviral drugs, there is still no cure or vaccine for HIV/AIDS—it is still a terminal illness.

## COPING AND TREATMENT

Receiving a diagnosis of HIV/AIDS brings emotional, financial, and social challenges. Medication treatment regimens can be complex and side effects can be severe.

There are clinics where health-care providers, social workers, and counselors can help make connections to other people or agencies that can assist an infected person with transportation, housing, childcare, employment, legal, and financial emergencies. According to the Mayo Clinic, these connections can help patients cope with living with HIV/AIDS.

Patients should educate themselves about HIV/AIDS. They should be active in their own care by researching how the disease usually progresses and learning about treatment options and their side effects.

Patients should build a strong support system. They can ask their family and friends for help; if they have problems dealing with the illness, they may seek to build relationships with a counselor, other people who are HIV-positive, or a support group.

Patients need to consider if they will keep their illness confidential or tell others about it. It may be difficult to reveal their illness to others, but they may eventually decide to confide in someone they trust.

---

**DID YOU KNOW?**

## AIDS Diagnoses by U.S. Region, 2001–2005

| | Regions | | | |
| --- | --- | --- | --- | --- |
| | South | Northeast | West | Midwest |
| Cases | 359,725 | 300,963 | 194,011 | 97,963 |

Whereas the highest number of AIDS cases existed in the South between 2001 and 2005, the fewest number of cases appeared in the Midwest.

Source: Centers for Disease Control and Prevention, Division of HIV/AIDS Prevention–Surveillance and Epidemiology; *HIV/AIDS Surveillance Report 2005*, Atlanta; U.S. Department of Health and Human Services, 2007.

---

They should tell any current and former sexual partners and their health-care providers.

Patients will benefit if they learn to accept the illness. This may be the hardest thing for someone to do, but there is a vast support network to help them cope with the disease. Some people rely on their faith for strength, others seek counselors with HIV experience, and others adopt a philosophy of living as fully as possible or helping others to deal with their illness.

*See also:* Cancer; Skin Disorders

**FURTHER READING**

Beck-Sague, Consuelo, and Caridad Beck. *Deadly Diseases and Epidemics: HIV/AIDS*. Philadelphia: Chelsea House, 2004.

DiSpezio, Michael A. *The Science, Spread, and Therapy of HIV Disease*. Shrewsbury, Mass.: ATL Press, 1998.

Ward, Darrell E. *The AmFAR AIDS Handbook*. New York: Norton, 1999.

# ■ ALCOHOLISM

An **addiction** to alcohol that includes a strong craving or compulsion to drink at regular intervals. Alcoholics lose control and generally cannot stop drinking after they have taken one drink. Because of their physical dependence on the drug, alcoholics experience withdrawal symptoms if they stop drinking. Physical dependence involves:

- a need for increasing amounts of alcohol to get drunk or achieve the desired effect;
- alcohol-related illnesses;
- blackouts, memory lapses after drinking;
- withdrawal symptoms when drinking stops.

## SYMPTOMS

Alcohol, a **depressant,** affects the central nervous system, resulting in decreases in activity, **anxiety,** inhibitions, and tension. Behavior, motor skills, and thinking are affected even after a few drinks. Impaired judgment and concentration and then drunkenness result.

Alcoholics can become skilled at covering up their problem so that even people close to them and people that see them every day are unaware of their drinking problems. Alcoholics also become expert manipulators of those around them, and those who fall prey to these manipulations and end up assisting the alcoholic to continue his or her habit are called **enablers.**

## STAGES OF ALCOHOLISM

The National Council on Alcoholism and Drug Dependence identifies four stages of the typical progression from alcohol use to addiction.

1. *Experimental stage*: Curious about alcohol's effects, the user tries alcohol one or more times;
2. *Social stage*: Alcohol is used occasionally in social situations such as parties or with friends;
3. *Dependent stage*: Obsessed with alcohol, the user consumes it regularly, often alone; and
4. *Chronic stage*: The user feels constant emotional or physical pain that is only reduced by alcohol.

## SYMPTOMS OF ALCOHOL WITHDRAWAL

When the brain has adapted to the alcohol and cannot function without it and alcohol is not available to it, alcohol withdrawal results. Symptoms are:

- anxiety
- **hallucinations** (seeing and hearing things that aren't there)
- increased blood pressure, heart rate, temperature, irregular heart rhythm

---

## DID YOU KNOW?

# Alcohol Abuse: Know the Signs

- abdominal pain, nausea, vomiting
- confusion
- drinking alone
- inability to stop or reduce alcohol intake
- morning drinking; shaking in the morning
- secretive behavior to hide alcohol use
- going to work or school drunk
- hostility when confronted about drinking
- drinking while taking prescribed and over-the-counter drugs that should not be taken while having alcohol in the bloodstream
- lying about drinking
- finding excuses to drink
- drinking more than intended
- drinking to fall asleep or escape problems
- having blackouts
- lost time due to sleeping off hangovers
- losing interest in schoolwork and career
- feeling tired much of the time
- neglecting to eat
- neglecting physical appearance
- avoiding nondrinking friends
- feeling more irritable; episodes of violence while drinking

  If you see signs of alcohol abuse in your own behavior, you should talk with an adult you trust about your drinking.

- loss of appetite, nausea, vomiting
- restlessness, nervousness
- seizures, tremors
- death (rarely)

**Delirium tremens (DTs)** is a severe form of alcohol withdrawal that involves sudden and severe mental or neurological changes and is a medical emergency requiring hospitalization. This is why alcoholics who decide to quit drinking usually go to a withdrawal facility, which will oversee the withdrawal and protect the person. Medication, monitoring, and intravenous fluids are usually required to prevent loss of life.

## RISK FACTORS

Scientists think the greatest risk factor for alcohol abuse is a family history of alcoholism. Determining whether it is a genetic factor that makes someone more susceptible to alcoholism or whether it is learned behavior from family members or both has long been the focus of much research. A majority of scientists have concluded that a family's genes are responsible for alcoholism in families. Studies of identical twins, who have identical DNA, show that if one is alcoholic, the other is most likely alcoholic as well. In addition, some children from alcoholic families, even when raised by nonalcoholic parents, have an increased risk for alcohol problems. However, the majority of people from families with a history of alcohol problems do *not* themselves become alcoholics.

In addition to genetic factors, having friends who abuse alcohol increases your risk of alcoholism. Relying on alcohol to escape problems at school and home and relieving anxiety puts one at risk for developing the disease. People who struggle with coping with normal challenges of life and who suffer from **depression** are at increased risk for dependence on alcohol. The age and circumstances at which a person starts drinking influences his or her future behavior. Because of their smaller size, children absorb alcohol into their bloodstream faster than would an older, larger person. Consequently, they become drunk sooner and stay drunk longer than would an adult. Alcohol's effect on a developing nervous system can be serious and lead to an addiction.

## SIGNS AND TESTS

A health-care provider will ask a person who is affected by alcohol questions about his or her drinking and family history.

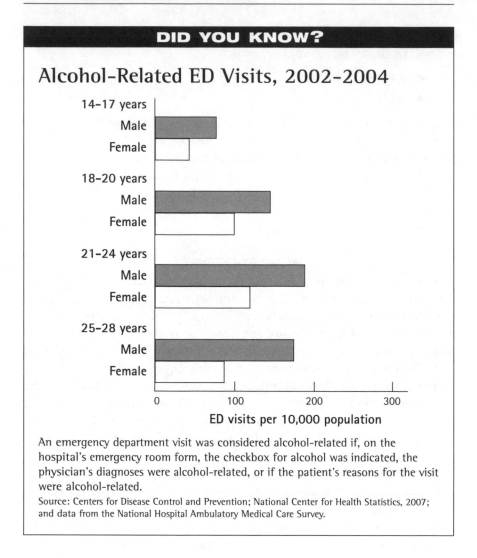

**DID YOU KNOW?**

# Alcohol-Related ED Visits, 2002–2004

ED visits per 10,000 population

An emergency department visit was considered alcohol-related if, on the hospital's emergency room form, the checkbox for alcohol was indicated, the physician's diagnoses were alcohol-related, or if the patient's reasons for the visit were alcohol-related.

Source: Centers for Disease Control and Prevention; National Center for Health Statistics, 2007; and data from the National Hospital Ambulatory Medical Care Survey.

The following questions are used by the National Institute on Alcohol Abuse and Alcoholism to screen people for alcohol abuse or dependence:

- Do you ever drive while drinking?
- Do you have to drink more than before to get drunk or feel the desired effect?
- Have you felt that you should cut down on your drinking?

- Have you ever had any blackouts after drinking?
- Have you ever missed work or lost a job because of drinking?
- Is someone in your family worried about your drinking?

## COPING AND TREATMENT

When people believe that their drinking may be out of control, trying to drink moderately can often be an effective way to deal with the problem. If moderation works, then the problem is solved. If not, the person may be ready to try **abstinence.** Those who are alcohol dependent need to stop drinking (abstinence) to recover from their addiction. The three steps of treatment are intervention, **detoxification,** and **rehabilitation.**

### Intervention

Research shows that compassion and empathy are more effective in helping people recognize they have an alcohol problem than is confrontation. Interventions are more successful if family and friends are honest with alcoholics about their concerns and help them realize that drinking is harming them.

### Detoxification

Detoxification, or withdrawal from alcohol, usually takes four to seven days if done in a controlled, supervised environment. A health-care provider will examine for liver and blood clotting problems and any other medical problems such as seizures. Vitamin supplements and a balanced diet are important as the body systems detoxify from alcohol. Delirium tremens (DTs) can be a complication as can depression or other mood disorders, and these can be identified and treated.

Disulfiram is a drug that causes the body to become very ill if alcohol is taken while on it. The behavioral aspect of anticipated symptoms is used to help prohibit an alcoholic from drinking.

Naltrexone is another type of drug used to help keep people addicted to alcohol or drugs to stay alcohol- and drug-free. It helps to block cravings for alcohol, and it blocks the effects of drugs that are opioids, including heroin, morphine, and cocaine. Patients take naltrexone once they have stopped drinking or taking drugs for at least five days, because if taken while alcohol or drugs are in the system, it will cause withdrawal symptoms. It must be taken carefully under the supervision of a doctor, as it has side effects and taking the wrong dose can be dangerous, especially to the liver.

A third type of drug is acamprosate, approved by the Food and Drug Administration in 2004. It helps to reverse the changes to the brain caused by drinking large amounts of alcohol. Acamprosate helps the recovering alcoholic to function normally after ceasing to drink, but it does not work if the person is still drinking. Health-care providers may decide to prescribe some combination of acamprosate, naltrexone, and disulfiram, depending on the needs of the individual patient.

### Rehabilitation

Rehabilitation programs can help people stay off alcohol after detoxification. Counseling, psychological support, medical care, and therapy involving education about alcoholism and its effects are available. Programs at rehabilitation centers can be inpatient or outpatient and are often partially staffed with recovering alcoholics who serve as role models. **Alcoholics Anonymous (AA)** is a self-help group of recovering alcoholics that offers emotional support and an abstinence model for those working on recovery from the disease. With local chapters throughout the United States, AA provides a recovery model, the 12-step approach, and help available 24 hours a day. Al-Anon is a support group for families and those affected by someone else's alcoholism; **Alateen** supports teenage children of alcoholics. Support groups with alternative approaches to the 12-step programs are also available.

### Success of Treatment Programs

Only 15 percent of people with alcohol dependence seek treatment for this disease. Resuming drinking again after treatment is common, so maintaining support systems to cope with slips and ensure that they do not turn into complete reversals is essential. Treatment programs have varying success rates, but many people with alcohol dependency make a full recovery.

## COMPLICATIONS OF ALCOHOLISM

Alcohol consumed during pregnancy can cause severe birth defects, the most serious being **fetal alcohol syndrome,** which can lead to mental retardation and behavior problems. A milder form of the condition that still causes lifelong problems is called fetal alcohol effects.

Alcohol is broken down and removed from the body by the liver. Over time, continued excess use of alcohol can develop into a network of scar tissue called **cirrhosis** of the liver. Irreversible liver failure as a result of chronic liver disease and cirrhosis is the 12th most common cause of death in the United States.

## SOCIAL AND ECONOMIC EFFECTS

Alcohol is a major social, economic, and public health problem. Alcohol is involved in more than half of all accidental deaths and almost half of all traffic deaths. A high percentage of suicides involve the use of alcohol along with other substances. People who use or are dependent on alcohol are more likely to be unemployed, involved in domestic violence, and have problems with the law, such as drinking and driving.

The National Institute on Alcohol Abuse and Alcoholism recommends that women have no more than one drink per day and men no more than two drinks per day. One drink is defined as a 12-ounce bottle of beer, a five-ounce glass of wine, or a 1½ ounce shot of liquor.

# TEENS SPEAK

## *My Struggle with Alcoholism*

I'm John and I'm an alcoholic. No, this isn't a line from a movie. It's my life.

At 14 I was angry. My parents had just divorced, and I ended up at a new school. I felt very unsure where I fit in. I got invited to a party at some kid's house, and there I had my first encounter with alcohol. I loved it—it gave me confidence and made the bad feelings go away for a little while.

Soon the weekend drinking—really bingeing—got worse and worse. I would drink anything, and in larger and larger amounts. Eventually I figured I could take a drink "for courage" to make it through the school day. I noticed if I went too long without a drink, I would get really anxious, get in fights, and even get shaky.

I hid it from my parents pretty well for a while. One day I was driving home after a party, and I ran the car off the road into someone's mailbox. I wasn't hurt, but the cops came and tested me for alcohol. Of course the level was really high. My parents blew a fuse, and I could tell they were really disappointed in me. They were working extra hard to make ends meet and trusting me to be responsible, and I did this.

I got sentenced to community service and rehab, since I had no priors and no one got hurt. My plan was to go through the motions, so I could get out and return to my life. Well, the first reality was going through detox. Because I was locked up and away from any alcohol, they put me on some medication so I didn't have seizures. It was still bad—I felt like jumping out of my skin. It was humiliating to realize my body was physically addicted at age 17 to alcohol—like some alcoholic. But I still didn't think I was one. I mean that's old guys, right?

I was struggling in the therapy sessions. They wanted me to talk about my life, how alcohol affected my life, my parents, and all that junk. I tried to survive by pushing in my feelings so I could just get through my time in rehab. Then one day, this 20-year-old guy came in—he would have been cool if not for the motorized wheelchair. As part of his sentence, he was here to tell us his story. He had been my age, 17, and pretty much doing the same thing—going out and drinking heavily on weekends, a little less during the week, and one day he had an accident. Only he killed someone else and changed a lot of lives. He killed a young father and broke his own neck so that he was permanently paralyzed. The genuine tears he had as he told of what he'd done and what it had done to all these other lives really got to me. He was me three years ago.

I actually opened up and let the counselors help me after that. I engaged in the therapy sessions and started going to Alcoholics Anonymous. It's got the best track record for keeping people sober. Going to their meetings and talking with other people who have been through what I have helps me keep up my resolve to stay sober and find other ways to have fun. So now I'm back finishing my last year of high school and planning to go to the community college next year. I'm playing baseball for fun, and I have found a different group of friends who enjoy life beyond the next party.

*See also:* Anxiety and Mood Disorders; Chronic Disease; Genetic Disorders; Heart Disease

**FURTHER READING**

Bellenir, Karen, ed. *Substance Abuse Sourcebook.* Detroit: Omnigraphics, 1996.
Stewart, Gail. *Teen Alcoholics.* San Diego, Calif.: Lucent, 2000.
Windle, Michael. *Alcohol Use Among Adolescents.* Thousand Oaks, Calif.: Sage, 1999.

# ■ ALLERGIES

A disorder in which the **immune system** is overly sensitive to a foreign substance not normally found in the human body. This foreign substance is called an **allergen.** Some examples of common allergens are pollen, dust, mold spores, pet dander (particles of animal skin, fur, or feathers), some foods, and even some medicines. Almost anything can be an allergen to an individual. The allergens get into the body when inhaled, eaten, or touched.

## SYMPTOMS AND CAUSES

If you have allergies, your immune system reacts to allergens by releasing chemicals known as **histamines.** Histamines are responsible for the symptoms of an allergy, such as sneezing, itching, swelling, mucus production, muscle spasms, hives, rashes, and watery eyes. There may be other symptoms as well, and they vary from person to person.

The symptoms you develop depend on the part of the body that the allergen contacts. Those that are breathed in often cause stuffy noses, itchy nose and throat, mucus production, cough, or wheezing. A food allergen can cause nausea, vomiting, abdominal pain, cramping, diarrhea, wheezing, or a severe, life-threatening reaction. Plant allergens often cause skin rashes. Drug allergies usually involve the whole body and can lead to a variety of symptoms.

## Severe Allergic Reactions

Severe allergic reactions to particular allergens can result in **anaphylactic shock,** which causes a massive release of histamine. In anaphylactic shock, the smooth muscles in the bronchioles contract, which restricts airflow into and out of the lungs.

Common allergens that cause severe allergic reactions are bee stings, penicillin, peanuts, and latex, which is used to make balloons and surgical gloves. People who are extremely sensitive to these allergens require prompt medical treatment if exposed to these agents because anaphylactic reactions are life-threatening. The reactions release histamines, which are powerful chemicals that can cause the throat to completely close from severe edema, or swelling of the tissues, in the throat and mouth.

## Allergy Testing

Allergy testing can determine whether symptoms are an actual allergy or caused by other problems. Skin testing is the most common method of allergy testing. One type of skin testing is the scratch test. It involves placing a small amount of the suspected allergy-causing substance on the skin and then slightly scratching the area so the substance moves under the skin. The skin is closely watched for signs of a reaction, which include swelling and redness. Another option is a blood test that measures levels of specific allergy-related substances. To test for medication or food allergies, yet another option is to avoid certain items to see if you get better, or to use suspected items to see if you feel worse. Your health-care provider may check your reaction to physical triggers by applying heat, cold, or other stimulation to the body and watching for an allergic response.

## PREVENTION AND TREATMENT

Once sensitivity to an allergen is diagnosed, avoiding the allergen is advised. Those who are allergic to pollen should avoid fields of tall grass; people allergic to dust can wash bedding frequently and use air filters and cleaners. The type and severity of symptoms determine what medications are prescribed. Sometimes, **antihistamines,** drugs that interfere with the action of histamines, may lessen the effect of the allergen. Short-acting antihistamines are available over the counter, and they help mild to moderate symptoms; more severe symptoms require prescriptions for longer acting antihistamines. Nasal sprays, allergy shots, and drugs that block specific allergens may also pro-

## DID YOU KNOW?

# Is It a Cold or an Allergy?

Although the symptoms, treatments, and complications for colds and allergies are similar, colds are caused by viruses, and allergies trigger the immune response.

| Symptoms | Cold | Airborne Allergy |
|---|---|---|
| Cough | Common | Sometimes |
| General aches, pains | Slight | Never |
| Fatigue, weakness | Sometimes | Sometimes |
| Itchy eyes | Rare or Never | Common |
| Sneezing | Usual | Usual |
| Sore throat | Common | Sometimes |
| Runny nose | Common | Common |
| Stuffy nose | Common | Common |
| Fever | Rare | Never |
| Duration | Three to 14 days | Weeks (for example, six weeks for ragweed or grass pollen seasons) |
| Treatment | Antihistamines Decongestants Nonsteroidal anti-inflammatory medicines | Antihistamines Nasal steroids Decongestants |
| Prevention | Wash your hands often; avoid close contact with anyone with a cold | Avoid those things that you are allergic to, such as pollen, dust, mites, mold, pet dander, cockroaches |
| Complications | Sinus infection Middle ear infection Asthma | Sinus infection Asthma |

Source: U.S. Department of Health and Human Services, National Institutes of Health, National Institute of Allergy and Infectious Diseases, 2005.

vide relief. For anaphylactic reactions, epinephrine can be lifesaving if given immediately.

# TEENS SPEAK

## How I Learned to Live with My Allergies

I'm Katie and I live with allergies. I've always had a tendency to sneeze, have drainage, and blow my nose. I really noticed it was bad when I was 13. It became my responsibility to mow the lawn at home, and it was just awful. It would take my older brother about an hour to get our yard done, but it was so much longer for me—like an hour and a half—because I had to keep stopping and sneezing.

So my parents took me to the pediatrician, and she sent me to an allergy specialist. Dr. Simons did allergy testing. She took these tiny racks of different potential allergens out. These were all things that are commonly known to cause allergies in many people. She stuck them on me, and it felt like a million little pricks on my back. It didn't hurt, it was just weird. Then I started itching in certain spots as I sat there. The doctor waited for several minutes to see which ones reacted.

It wasn't surprising that I was allergic to grass, but I was surprised to learn I had other allergies too. Pollen, cats, dust, and different trees made a large bump indicating I was allergic to them too. So the allergist made a solution that had small amounts of these things. I soon began weekly allergy shots. The nurse gave them, and it really didn't hurt because the needle was so small. The skin around it would itch and sometimes get a little red. Over time the shots would get me used to these allergens so my immune system would quit responding to them as foreign bodies to fight against.

It took some time to notice a change—probably a year or two. But I did start to be able to be outdoors without sneezing every time. In the meantime, I used drugs called antihistamines. These drugs fight the histamine release that occurs when your body perceives an allergen as an invading foreign body. They stop the sneezing and runny nose symptoms for several hours. Some kinds of antihistamines have the side effect of sleepiness, which makes it hard for some people to tolerate them. I had that problem with a couple of kinds but did okay with another brand. Now that I'm 16, the shots are every other week, and the nurse taught my mom to give me the shots.

I never had problems with breathing like my friend Suzie. She has allergies too, but she starts wheezing and can't breathe so well. She was diagnosed with asthma caused by allergies. So, she had to start inhalers in addition to the allergy shots and antihistamines. She's doing better now that she's on her medicine too. It no longer affects our lives so much. We both are in band and just finished band camp—with all the pollen and grass—without any problems. The doctor is hopeful that the injections and time will make it so I no longer have to take allergy shots or medications to control my symptoms.

*See also:* Skin Disorders

**FURTHER READING**
Briner, William. *Action Plan for Allergies*. Champaign, Ill.: Human Kinetics, 2006.
Kwong, Frank K., with Bruce Cook. *The Complete Allergy Book*. Naperville, Ill.: Sourcebooks, 2002.

# ■ ALZHEIMER'S DISEASE AND DEMENTIA

A progressive brain disease in which brain cells are damaged and proteins accumulate abnormally in the brain. As many as 5 million Americans have Alzheimer's, which causes problems with memory, thinking, and behavior severe enough to impact their work and social lives. The seventh-leading cause of death in the United States, Alzheimer's accounts for between 50 and 70 percent of **dementia** cases. Dementia is a loss of memory and other mental abilities severe enough to interfere with daily life.

## SYMPTOMS

Although some changes in memory are normal as people age, the symptoms of those with Alzheimer's are more than simple memory loss. Alzheimer's causes problems with reasoning, thinking, learning, and communicating. The problems impact work, socializing, and family life.

The Alzheimer's Association lists these warning signs of the disease: memory loss including forgetting recently learned information; difficulty performing familiar tasks; language problems including forgetting simple words and substituting unusual words; becoming disoriented in time and place—forgetting where they are and how to get back home; exercising poor judgment; having problems with abstract thinking; misplacing things; changes in mood, behavior, and personality; and becoming more passive. A health-care provider can distinguish between Alzheimer's and the normal expression of these characteristics.

# Fact Or Fiction?

### Alzheimer's disease is not fatal.

**The Facts:** Alzheimer's disease does cause death by destroying brain cells. It causes memory changes, irregular behaviors, and loss of body functions. It slowly erodes one's identity, ability to form relationships, think, eat, talk, and walk, and it eventually leads to death.

## RISK FACTORS

Increasing age is the greatest known risk factor for Alzheimer's, and most people with the disease are 65 or older. Every five years after age 65 the risk for the disease doubles; after age 85 the risk is nearly 50 percent. Research also shows **genes** play a role in Alzheimer's. If a parent, brother, sister, or child has Alzheimer's, one is more likely to develop Alzheimer's. The probability of getting the disease increases if more than one family member has the disease.

Behaviors that will reduce your risk of having Alzheimer's disease are protecting yourself from serious head injury by using seat belts and sports helmets; avoiding falls; keeping your heart and blood vessels healthy and avoiding high blood pressure, heart disease, stroke, diabetes, and high **cholesterol**; keeping your brain and social connections healthy; maintaining healthy weight; and avoiding tobacco use and excess alcohol intake.

## TREATMENT

Currently there is no cure for Alzheimer's, but there are services and support for coping with the symptoms. In some cases, drugs may slow the development of the disease, but it eventually progresses. There is an ongoing worldwide effort to find better ways to treat the disease, delay its onset, and prevent its development.

*See also:* Alcoholism; Diabetes Mellitus (DM); Genetic Disorders; Heart Disease

### FURTHER READING

Hains, Bryan. *Brain Disorders*. Philadelphia: Chelsea House, 2006.
Shankle, William Rodman, and Daniel G. Amen. *Preventing Alzheimer's*.
New York: Putnam, 2004.

# ■ ANEMIA

A common blood disorder in which the part of the blood that carries oxygen is abnormal. **Hemoglobin** is the part of red blood cells that absorbs oxygen from the lung tissues and carries it to the body cells. In a person with anemia, there is either not enough hemoglobin in the blood or the hemoglobin is defective.

At first, anemia can go undetected because the signs and symptoms are so mild, but they increase as the condition progresses. The main symptom of most types of anemia is fatigue, which can be accompanied by a fast or irregular heartbeat, dizziness, headache, weakness, shortness of breath, numbness or coldness in extremities, pale skin, or chest pain. Some types of anemia can cause feelings of numbness and tingling in the extremities, called neuropathy, and sometimes a person with anemia will crave ice or certain foods.

# Q & A

**Question: Is constant craving and chewing of ice a sign of anemia?**

**Answer:** It could be. Craving and chewing ice is often associated with iron deficiency anemia, although it can also be a sign of other problems. Pica is the term for craving and chewing substances such as ice or paper that provide no nutrition.

Scientists do not know why some people with iron deficiency anemia crave and chew ice. Some research suggests it could be due to the pain-relieving property of ice that helps the people who suffer from iron deficiency anemia with tongue pain and **inflammation.** The same research found that ice has a different and better taste to people with anemia than to others without anemia.

## CAUSES

Floating in **plasma,** the liquid part of the blood, are three types of cells—white blood cells, platelets, and red blood cells. The red blood cells contain an iron-rich protein, hemoglobin, which enables them to carry oxygen to all parts of the body. Produced regularly in the bone marrow, the red blood cells and hemoglobin are made of iron, protein, and vitamins from food. Anemia results from a below-normal number of red blood cells or below-normal hemoglobin within red blood cells.

### Common Types of Anemia and Their Causes

Iron deficiency anemia is the most common type. Without enough iron, the body does not produce enough hemoglobin for red blood cells. Usually the iron in dead blood cells is recycled into new blood cells, so if you lose blood, you lose iron. Menstruation can cause women who lose a lot of blood each month to be at risk of iron deficiency anemia. Iron deficiency anemia can also be caused by a **chronic** blood loss from conditions such as ulcers or colon cancer. An iron-poor diet or a growing fetus in a pregnant woman can lead to iron loss and iron deficiency anemia.

Vitamin deficiency anemias may be caused by a diet lacking **folate** and vitamin B12 or other key nutrients. Not getting enough of these nutrients can cause a decrease in production of red blood cells. People who have disorders of the intestines can develop this type of anemia.

Chronic diseases can cause anemia. Cancer, Crohn's disease, and rheumatoid arthritis are examples of chronic inflammatory diseases that interfere with the production of red blood cells and cause chronic anemia. Kidney failure can also cause chronic anemia. **Chemotherapy,** radiation therapy, environmental toxins, pregnancy, and lupus are all thought to be possible causes of aplastic anemia, a life-threatening anemia caused by the inability to produce all three types of blood cells.

Sickle-cell anemia is inherited mainly by people of African and Arabic descent. In this anemia, the red blood cells have a crescent (sickle) shape caused by a defective form of hemoglobin. The sickle-shaped cells die prematurely, which results in a chronic shortage of red blood cells. The sickle cells can also cause pain if they block blood from flowing through small blood vessels of the body.

## RISK FACTORS

Factors that increase the risk of anemia are poor diet, intestinal disorders, menstruation, pregnancy, chronic conditions, and family history of anemia. People with diabetes, people dependent on alcohol, and strict vegetarians who may not get enough iron or vitamin B12 in their diets are also at risk.

## PREVENTION

Eating a healthful, varied diet, including iron-rich foods, folate, and vitamin B12, can help you avoid anemia. Beef and other meats are good sources of iron, as are beans, lentils, iron-fortified cereals, dark green leafy vegetables, dried fruit, nuts, and seeds. Folate and folic acid are found in citrus juices and fruits, dark green leafy vegetables, legumes, and fortified breakfast cereals. Meat and dairy products contain vitamin B12. Citrus fruits and other foods containing vitamin C help increase iron absorption. Infants and children, pregnant and menstruating women, strict vegetarians, and long-distance runners have high iron requirements and should eat plenty of iron-rich foods.

## TREATMENT

Treatments for anemia are based on the causes. Sometimes health-care providers prescribe iron or folic acid supplements if a healthy diet does not provide adequate amounts. Other treatments are surgery for chronic blood losses, injections of vitamin B12, blood transfusions to boost red blood cell levels, and even bone marrow transplantation for anemias connected to bone marrow disease. Treatments for sickle-cell anemia can include oxygen, pain relieving drugs, fluids to reduce pain, blood transfusions, folic acid supplements, and **antibiotics**. In some cases, a bone marrow transplant or cancer medication is prescribed.

# TEENS SPEAK

## *Keisha Talks About Sickle-Cell Anemia*

I want to tell you about living with sickle-cell anemia [sickle cell disease]. I'm 17, and I've been hospitalized five times in my life for what they call sickle-cell crisis. I found out about it when I was 10, and I became very short of breath and soon after was in awful pain. My parents took me to the emergency room. I was admitted to the hospital, and they did a lot of tests on me. It turns out that my parents, who are both healthy, are carriers of the sickle-cell gene, and I was born with the genetic trait.

My parents and the nurses made sure to teach me as much as I could handle, and I remember that first picture of a red blood cell that is curved in half. When I'm in crisis, it's hard for me to believe that little curve in a little cell could be the cause of this awful pain.

Most of the time, I'm a high school junior who is as normal as anyone else. But I can have some outside or internal stress hit me that affect the cell shapes. Before I know it, I'm in terrible pain—my back, my abdomen, my arms, and legs. And my breathing is not very good when this happens.

I end up having to go to the ER and getting IV fluids and transfusions. They do give me pain medication so the pain is tolerable, but it doesn't go away right away. After a few days of therapy, they stop the IVs and the blood and the oxygen, and I no longer need the pain medication. Then I'm discharged back home.

I get frustrated that I can't really prevent this from coming on and it can ruin events I've anticipated. I have to be out of school when this happens, and I always have to catch up. I want to go to college and need good grades, so I can't get behind.

It's doubtful I will have children. Right now that's not a big deal, but my parents think I'll have issues when I'm older and find someone to marry. Even if I could go through the physical stress, I do not want to pass on the trait to children knowing what I know and knowing there is no cure for this.

*See also:* Alcoholism; Chronic Disease; Diabetes Mellitus (DM); Genetic Disorders

**FURTHER READING**

Harris, Jacqueline. *Sickle-Cell Disease.* Brookfield, Conn.: Twenty-First Century Books, 2001.

Mayo Clinic. Diseases and Conditions: Anemia. URL: www.mayoclinic.com/health/anemia/ds00321. Accessed July 15, 2008.

# ■ ANXIETY AND MOOD DISORDERS

Lasting at least six months, **anxiety** disorders cause people to have prolonged fearfulness and uncertainty. Everyone experiences anxiety when he or she face a stressful event such as public speaking, but anxiety disorders last much longer and, if they remain untreated, they can get worse.

About 40 million American adults, or about 18 percent, suffer from anxiety disorders every year. Other mental or physical illnesses, including alcohol or substance abuse, often accompany anxiety disorders, and these other illnesses may need to be treated before a person can be treated for the anxiety disorder. There are a number of anxiety disorders, each with different symptoms, but all the symptoms cluster around excessive, irrational fear and dread. Anxiety disorders include panic disorder, obsessive-compulsive disorder, **post-traumatic stress disorder (PTSD)**, social anxiety disorder, specific phobia, and **generalized anxiety disorder.**

**Depression** and **bipolar disorder** are mood disorders in which people experience abnormal moods for the situations they experience. Their moods make people with these illnesses unable to concentrate on school, sports, or friends. Preoccupied, they cannot make changes in their lives to change their moods. The symptoms of mood disorders continue unless they are treated.

## PANIC DISORDER

One type of anxiety disorder is panic disorder. Symptoms of panic disorder are sudden terror attacks, a pounding heart, sweatiness, weakness, faintness and dizziness, numbness in hands, nausea, chest pain, or sensations of smothering. Fear of losing control, a belief one is having a heart attack or losing one's mind, and near-death feelings usually accompany attacks. Although the attacks generally peak within 10 minutes, symptoms of an attack can last much longer. Not everyone who has panic attacks will develop panic disorder; some people have only one attack.

Repeated panic attacks can disable people so that they start to avoid places or situations where their attacks have occurred. The lives of people with panic disorders can become so restricted that they avoid normal activities, such as grocery shopping or driving. One-third become housebound. This condition is called agoraphobia, or fear of open spaces.

In most cases, people with panic disorder respond to medication and/or **psychotherapy** to change thinking patterns that lead to anxiety. Depression, drug abuse, or alcoholism often accompany panic disorder. Symptoms of depression include sadness, inability to enjoy activities, hopelessness, changes in sleep and appetite, low energy, difficulty in concentrating, and thoughts of death or suicide. Usually, **antidepressants** and/or psychotherapy can effectively treat depression.

### OBSESSIVE-COMPULSIVE DISORDER (OCD)

People with obsessive-compulsive disorder (OCD) control anxiety produced by persistent (obsessive) thoughts by using rituals (compulsions). In OCD, the rituals end up controlling them. An example of OCD is people obsessed with germs who compulsively wash their hands over and over. Performing the ritual relieves the anxiety created by their obsessive thoughts. Other common rituals are counting things, sequentially touching things, or being preoccupied with order and symmetry.

Performing these rituals interferes with the daily lives of the 2.2 million American adults who are affected by OCD; one-third of adults with OCD develop symptoms as children. Accompanying OCD can be eating disorders, other anxiety disorders, or depression. Symptoms of OCD may disappear and then come back, or they may get worse, or get better over time. Severe OCD can affect people's work and impact their handling of home responsibilities as they try to avoid the triggers of their obsessions. Certain medications and psychotherapy may successfully treat people with OCD.

### POST-TRAUMATIC STRESS DISORDER (PTSD)

Post-traumatic stress disorder (PTSD) develops after a terrifying experience involving physical harm or threat of physical harm. PTSD sufferers have experienced traumatic events such as war, rape, mugging, torture, kidnappings, child abuse, plane crashes, bombing, and natural disasters. People with PTSD startle easily, become emotionally numb, lose interest in things they used to enjoy, and become irritable, aggressive, and even violent. They avoid situations reminding them of the traumatic event. They have flashbacks in which they relive the trauma of the event during the day and in nightmares.

Symptoms must last more than a month to be considered PTSD; symptoms usually begin within three months of the traumatic incident but can occur years afterward. The disorder affects about 7.7 million American adults, but it can occur at any age. Some evidence suggests that a tendency to develop the disorder is inherited. Medication and psychotherapy are used to treat the symptoms.

## SOCIAL ANXIETY DISORDER

Social anxiety disorder, also called social phobia, is an illness in which people become overwhelmingly anxious and self-conscious in everyday social situations. Symptoms include intense, persistent, and **chronic** fear of being watched and judged by others and of doing embarrassing things. People with social anxiety disorder can worry for days or weeks before a dreaded situation. When severe, the condition can interfere with work, school, and other ordinary activities and can make it difficult to make and keep friends.

Physical symptoms of social anxiety disorder are blushing, profuse sweating, trembling, nausea, and difficulty speaking. Other anxiety disorders, depression, or substance abuse may accompany the disease, which about 15 million American adults have. Psychotherapy and medications are used in treatment.

## SPECIFIC PHOBIA

Specific phobia is an intense, irrational fear of something that in reality poses little or no threat. Some common specific phobias are heights, escalators, tunnels, highway driving, closed-in places, water, flying, dogs, spiders, and blood. **Agoraphobia** is an example of a specific phobia in which one fears open spaces or going outside the home. When people have to face their phobias, they may have panic attacks and severe anxiety. People with specific phobias respond to carefully targeted psychotherapy.

## GENERALIZED ANXIETY DISORDER (GAD)

Generalized anxiety disorder (GAD) causes people to go through the day filled with worry and tension, although there is nothing to cause it. They are overly concerned with health, money, family issues, and work difficulties as they anticipate disaster. GAD is diagnosed when a person worries excessively about a variety of everyday problems for at least six months. Although they may realize they are more anxious than their situation warrants, they are unable to stop worrying. Unable to relax, they startle easily and have difficulty concentrating. Accompanying symptoms may be sleeplessness, fatigue, headaches, muscle tension, muscle aches, difficulty swallowing, twitching, irritability, sweating, nausea, lightheadedness, feeling out of breath, and hot flashes. If their anxiety level is mild, people with GAD can function socially and have a job. Other people may have difficulty carrying out the simplest daily activities. GAD affects about 6.8 million American adults and may be inherited. Accompanying GAD may be other anxiety disorders, depression, or substance abuse. Medication and psychotherapy are commonly used for treatment.

# TEENS SPEAK

## *I Live with Generalized Anxiety Disorder*

I was about 15 when I was diagnosed with generalized anxiety disorder. GAD came on over time. At first I noticed I couldn't sleep like I used to—I would wake up at 3:30 every morning with my mind racing and thinking about some stupid thing. I couldn't get it out of my mind and I couldn't relax enough to go back to sleep. So I'd lay there for a while and toss and turn. Of course, I was tired and irritable during the day and the slightest thing could make me cry. And I would worry about the slightest thing like it was a big deal.

As time went on, I felt more and more jittery and sometimes my heart would race and I'd feel lightheaded. My mom took me to my nurse practitioner and she evaluated me. I had a physical and lab work done, but everything came back normal. She asked me a lot of questions about my stress and depression and even gave me a couple written tests. I found out that I had generalized anxiety disorder and it's very easy to treat in most people. Although many people also have depression, I did not. I felt so relieved to know there was something that could be done to make me feel better.

The nurse practitioner set me up with a psychologist to talk about how I was feeling and to learn to rethink how I see things so I don't get so jumpy at every little thing. She also prescribed an antidepressant because those have been shown to work at helping GAD. Actually about a week or two after I started the medicine I felt much calmer, and I have slept through the night since then and can cope with everyday things again. I will have to take the medicine for a year or more before we see if I can come off it without having my symptoms return. I only needed a few sessions with the psychologist and I can just call if I need to see him again.

## DEPRESSION

Depression is a disabling mood disorder characterized by a low mood that affects a person's feelings, thoughts, behaviors, and physical well-being for months or even years. When they are diagnosing depression, most health-care providers look for at least five of the following criteria during the same two-week period: depressed mood most of the day nearly every day; less pleasure in almost all activities nearly every day; significant weight gain or loss not due to dieting; insomnia or increased sleeping; abnormal speeding up or slowing down of activities and thinking nearly every day; fatigue or loss of energy; feelings of worthlessness or excessive guilt, difficulty in thinking, concentrating, or making decisions; and thoughts of death. In addition to five of the previous symptoms, at least the first or second symptom must also be present; it cannot be simply a normal reaction to a loved one's death.

Depression affects more Americans than AIDS, cancer, and heart failure combined. One in 10 people will experience depression at some point in life. For a long time, mental health-care providers thought that depression was only an illness of adults. In the 1990s, research showed that young people do indeed develop serious depressive disorders in adolescence. In the United States, one in 10 teenagers experiences major depression every year. In 2005, 2.2 million teens, or 9 percent of the teen population, experienced major depression. Between the ages of 12 and 17, the risk of depression increases greatly; 16- and 17-year-olds have a 30 percent higher rate of depression than that of other adolescents.

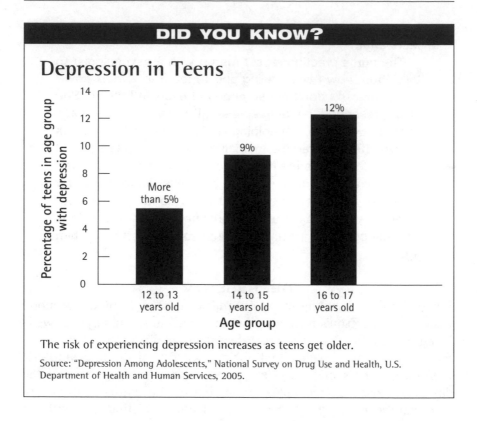

**DID YOU KNOW?**

## Depression in Teens

The risk of experiencing depression increases as teens get older.

Source: "Depression Among Adolescents," National Survey on Drug Use and Health, U.S. Department of Health and Human Services, 2005.

There is a gender gap in regard to depression. In 12- to 17-year-olds, 5 percent of boys and 13 percent of girls have depression. Women are diagnosed with depression twice as often as men. It is possible that men seek treatment less often or that they are more likely to "self-medicate" with alcohol or drugs.

Researchers have found that if you have one parent with depression, you have a 25 percent higher chance of having it also. If both parents have depression, your risk increases to 75 percent. In addition to heredity, chemical imbalances can contribute to depression. The brain constantly makes **neurotransmitters** and hormones, which are important chemicals that transfer information and instructions from the brain to the body about energy, growth, sleep, digestion, hunger, happiness, and self-esteem. Stresses, such as life changes, social problems, abuse, or trauma can contribute to neurotransmitter imbalances which then cause the symptoms of depression. The medications that are used in depression treatment impact the neurotransmitter imbalances that affect people's feelings.

## Depression and Other Illness

People with depression have more physical illnesses and require more health-care services than those without the illness. One theory about the cause of the increased physical illness is that depression may suppress the **immune system.** Depression can also lead to unhealthy behaviors such as the use of drugs and alcohol. Because it is a **depressant,** alcohol makes depression worse. A 2004 U.S. Department of Health and Human Services study shows that teens with depression are twice as likely to use alcohol, cigarettes, and drugs as those who do not have depression.

## Importance of Treatment of Teen Depression

Although depression is a treatable disease, fewer than half the teenagers who experience it seek treatment. If left untreated, over time the symptoms of depression can take a significant toll on the functioning and development of teens. Additionally, suicide is the third leading cause of death in adolescents and successful treatment can reduce this rate.

Research shows that a combination of psychotherapy and prescription medication is the most effective treatment for depression. The psychotherapist can help the depressed person understand and change negative thoughts and behavior patterns. People also benefit from therapy's help in becoming more aware of their problems and learning what triggers their depression. Cognitive-behavioral therapy (CBT) is a form of psychotherapy that focuses on thoughts (cognition) and on behavior. CBT can help people change the way they think about themselves and their problems. For example, people whose depression makes them think they have to achieve impossible goals can learn to set realistic ones. Research from 2004 reported in the *Journal of the American Medical Association* showed that 71 percent of people treated for depression with a combination of medication and CBT had a reduction in symptoms.

Exercise is often recommended for those suffering from depression. Many people experience a "runner's high" or a surge of neurotransmitters that make them feel in a happier mood after aerobic exercise. The side effects of exercise (distraction from worry, support from team members, self-esteem boost from reaching a goal) can also positively affect people's moods. Other forms of treatment include support groups and self-help groups in which members share information and strategies for coping with depression; meditation, which helps

## Treatment for Depression in Teens

| Age Group | Percentage of Teens with Depression Who Receive Treatment |
|---|---|
| 12 to 13 years old | 40 percent receive treatment |
| 14 to 15 years old | 30 percent receive treatment |
| 16 to 17 years old | 45 percent receive treatment |

Although 80 percent of people seeking treatment for depression are treated successfully, fewer than half of the teens with depression receive treatment.

Source: "Depression among Adolescents," National Survey on Drug Use and Health, U.S. Department of Health and Human Services, 2005.

one focus on the present rather than worries about the past or future; and acupuncture, the Chinese practice of using needles to rebalance energy flow that is out of balance.

If you have friends or family with depression, you can help them cope with the illness by just being with them and helping them know they are not alone; by not expecting that your being overly cheerful will solve their problems; and by trying to not be angry or blaming.

### BIPOLAR DISORDER

A brain disorder also known as manic-depressive illness that causes unusual shifts in a person's mood, energy, and ability to function. Everyone has ups and downs in mental outlook, but the symptoms of bipolar disorder are severe. Poor performance in schools and jobs, relationship problems, and even suicide can result. With treatment, however, people with the disorder can live full, productive lives.

Most people with bipolar disorder develop symptoms in late adolescence or early adulthood; some develop their first symptoms in childhood, and some later in life. Bipolar disorder causes dramatic mood swings from "high" and/or irritable to sad and hopeless, and then back again, often with normal mood periods between. Periods of highs are episodes of **mania.**

Mania episode symptoms can include increased energy, activity, and restlessness, excessively "high" mood, extreme irritability, racing thoughts, distractibility, no need for sleep, poor judgment, spending sprees, abuse of drugs (especially cocaine, alcohol, and sleeping medications), and aggressive behavior.

Symptoms of the depressive episode include lasting sad, anxious, or empty moods; feelings of hopelessness, pessimism, feelings of guilt, worthlessness, or helplessness; loss of interest or pleasure in activities, decreased energy, fatigue, difficulty concentrating and remembering, restlessness, too much or no sleep, change in appetite, and thoughts of death. The diagnosis of bipolar disorder is made based on symptoms, course of illness, and family history.

The disorder runs in families, so researchers are searching for specific **genes** that increase a person's chance of becoming bipolar. New brain imaging techniques help scientists to learn about the way the brain of a person with bipolar disorder differs from the brain of a person without the disorder.

A combination of mood stabilizing medications and psychosocial treatment (including psychotherapy) helps people manage the disorder over time. Therapy can help people with bipolar disorder change negative thought patterns and behaviors, learn the signs of relapse, reduce the level of stress in their families, improve personal relationships, and regulate their daily schedules to protect against manic episodes.

# Q & A

**Question: When friends or family members have bipolar disorder, how can a person cope with the stress of their unpredictable behavior?**

**Answer:** When friends or family members have mild bipolar disorder, their moods may flip-flop from sad to irritable, excited to indifferent, or affectionate to aloof, and friends and family may never know what to expect or how to help them. Joining a support group or going to family counseling may help one understand the disease and plan effective ways of coping with the stress.

## SUICIDE

Most people who commit suicide have a mental or emotional disorder, usually depression. Thirty to 70 percent of suicide victims

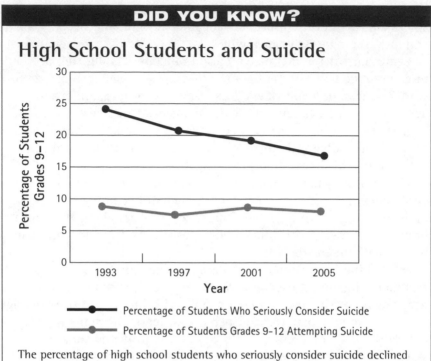

# High School Students and Suicide

The percentage of high school students who seriously consider suicide declined between 1993 and 2005 from 24.1 percent to 16.9 percent, although the percentage of students who have attempted suicide has not declined as much.

Source: Centers for Disease Control and Prevention, 2007.

have major depression or bipolar disorder. The signals that someone needs help and is in serious trouble include expressing in words that he or she is thinking about suicide ("Maybe I won't be around" or "You'd be better off without me"), and showing changes in personality and lack of interest in future plans. They might also express hopelessness or helplessness, and they might give away their prized possessions. Having depression and undertaking risky or daring behaviors are other signals. Any one of the signals does not mean that the person will attempt suicide, but several of them might be a call for help.

According to the Centers for Disease Control in 2006, suicide is the 11th leading cause of death in the United States. In the past 60 years, the adolescent suicide rate has tripled, making it the third leading cause of death among 15- to 24-year-olds and the second leading cause of death among college students.

**DID YOU KNOW?**

## Suicide on Campus

|  | Women | Men | Total |
|---|---|---|---|
| Very sad | 55.5 percent | 41.9 percent | 50.3 percent |
| Hopeless | 36.5 percent | 28.3 percent | 33.4 percent |
| So depressed could not function | 24 percent | 19 percent | 22.1 percent |
| Seriously considered suicide | 9.9 percent | 9.5percent | 9.7 percent |
| Attempted suicide | 1.4 percent | 1.6 percent | 1.5 percent |

Much higher percentages of college women than college men report feeling very sad, hopeless, or so depressed that they could not function. However, slightly more men than women attempt suicide.

Source: American College Health Association, 2001.

Eight out of 10 suicidal persons give some sign of their intentions. Research shows that people who threaten to commit suicide, talk about it, or call suicide crisis lines are 30 times more likely than average to kill themselves. Nearly three-fourths of suicide victims visit a

**DID YOU KNOW?**

## College Students Considering Suicide

- While 6.8 percent of college women consider suicide **1 to 2 times,** a lower percentage of men—5.4 percent—consider suicide 1 to 2 times.
- While 3.1 percent of college women consider suicide **3 to 4 times,** a higher percentage of men—3.3 percent—consider suicide more often.

Although a higher percentage of college women consider suicide once or twice, more college men than women consider it three to four times—in other words, more often.

Source: American College Health Association, 2001.

doctor in the four months prior to their deaths, and half of them visit a doctor in the month before.

Trusting your instincts about someone in trouble and talking with him or her about your concerns is important, as is listening to what the person has to say. Try to remain nonjudgmental as you determine whether he or she has a plan; the more detailed the plan, the higher the risk. Rather than counseling the person, try to enlist professional help, but do not leave the person alone.

People who are considering suicide may drink alcohol in hopes that it will make them feel better. However, studies indicate that alcohol, as well as previously attempting suicide, is often a factor in suicide. According to 2007 Mental Health America statistics, 40 percent of suicide victims made a previous attempt; 50 percent of suicides are instigated by alcohol; and alcohol abusers comprise 20 percent of suicides.

No one treatment approach is appropriate for all suicidal persons. Medication, talk therapy, or a combination is the most commonly used. Talk (cognitive) therapy and behavioral therapies get suicidal people thinking in new ways about themselves and the world and train them in problem solving, social skills, and relaxation, with the goal of reducing anxiety and depression. The therapist emphasizes that the client is doing most of the work so that the suicidal person does not see the therapist as essential for survival.

Medications treat the depression associated with suicide. Antidepressants affect the mood-related chemical pathways of the brain. Two of the most common types of antidepressants are selective serotonin reuptake inhibitors (SSRIs) and tricyclic antidepressants (TCAs). Doctors also prescribe an older drug, monoamine oxidase inhibitors (MAOIs). Three newer types of antidepressants used are alpha-2 antagonists, serotonin and **norepinephrine** reuptake inhibitors (SNRIs), and aminoketones. Through consistent monitoring of drug reactions, doctors can prescribe the most effective treatment for depression with the fewest side effects. The doctor will take into consideration all other medications that the person takes in order to avoid dangerous interactions and will advise the person about the dangers of having alcohol and other drugs while on antidepressants.

A week or two following the start of medication, insomnia may lessen or disappear; three or four weeks can bring an improvement in mood; and in six to eight weeks of treatment, the full benefits of the medication may take effect. Changes in amount and types of medications may need to take place, and, once the depression has improved it is recommended taking the medications another four to nine months. If the depression is chronic, the patient may need to continue the medication beyond that to avoid recurring episodes.

In 2001, Surgeon General David Satcher, M.D., Ph.D., announced the first national suicide prevention strategy. The plan, *The National Strategy for Suicide Prevention: Goals and Objectives for Action,* aims to prevent premature deaths due to suicide, reduce rates of suicidal behaviors, reduce traumatic effects of suicide on family and friends, and promote resources, respect, and interconnectedness for individuals, families, and communities.

*See also:* Alcoholism; Eating Disorders; Genetic Disorders; Obesity; Treatment

**FURTHER READING**

Castle, Lana. *Bipolar Disorder Demystified.* New York: Marlowe, 2003.

Connolly, Sucheta, David Simpson, and Cynthia Petty. *Anxiety Disorders.* Philadelphia: Chelsea House, 2006.

Moehn, Heather. *Coping with Social Anxiety.* New York: Rosen, 2001.

# ARTHRITIS

A group of diseases that may cause pain, stiffness, and swelling in the joints and in areas close to the joints. Joints are places in the body where two bones meet. Because it is a chronic disease (affecting someone over a long period of time), arthritis comes in many forms. Some forms appear, disappear, and return later; others appear gradually.

Arthritis can appear in any body joint; it can be triggered by injury, lack of physical activity, wear and tear on the joints, or genetics. There are three types of arthritis most common in older adults.

## OSTEOARTHRITIS

Osteoarthritis is the most common form of arthritis and is one of the major causes of physical disability among older people. By age 65, more than half the population of the United States has evidence of osteoarthritis in at least one joint. It affects hands, the lower back, the neck, and joints such as knees, hips, and feet, but does not affect internal organs. Symptoms range from mild pain and stiffness to severe pain in joints. Osteoarthritis is caused when the cartilage at the ends of bones breaks down and wears away so the bones rub against each other causing pain, swelling, and loss of motion in the joint. Too much stress on a previously injured joint, misalignment of joints, and excess weight may increase risk of developing osteoarthritis. Treatment plans often include exercise, rest and joint care, pain relief, weight control, medicines, surgery, and nontraditional treatment approaches.

Early treatment is aimed at exercise, weight loss, appropriate joint rest and care during acute pain, and medication such as acetamino-phen, aspirin, nonsteroidal anti-inflammatory drugs, and the newer COX-2 inhibitors. When the pain is unable to be controlled with medication or the joint is so degraded that movement is poor, joint replacement is usually the surgical treatment undertaken.

## Q & A

**Question: How can exercising a hip or knee with arthritis manage or reduce pain instead of making it worse?**

**Answer:** Improving muscle tone around the joint actually protects and stabilizes it. If the joint is allowed to become more unstable, it will make more osteoarthritis. People with osteoarthritis of the hip and knee can best exercise by walking, bicycling, or, especially, swimming, which uses the water's buoyancy to assist in motion and doesn't put weight on the joints. Jogging is not recommended for people with osteoarthritis due to the extreme weight load it puts on joints.

### RHEUMATOID ARTHRITIS

Rheumatoid arthritis may affect the skin, lungs, eyes, and blood vessels, as well as the joints, causing people to feel sick, tired, and sometimes feverish. Usually beginning during a person's most productive years (ages 20–50), rheumatoid arthritis involves the **immune system's** mistaking the body's own healthy cells and tissues as invaders and attacking them. Rheumatoid arthritis results from such interacting factors as **genes, hormones,** and the environment. Some research shows that **infectious** agents such as **viruses** and **bacteria** can trigger rheumatoid arthritis in people with the genes for developing the disease; the specific agents for causing the disease are not yet known. Treatment plans can include exercise, medication, stress reduction, and, in some cases, surgery.

## GOUT

The third most common form of arthritis, gout, causes sudden intense pain and swelling in the joints, usually the joints in the lower parts of the body such as the ankles, heels, knees, or toes, which can also be red and warm. Frequently occurring at night, attacks can be triggered by stressful events, alcohol, certain drugs, or another disease. Early attacks usually last between three and 10 days, and the next attack may be months or years afterward. The buildup of needlelike uric acid crystals in connective tissue and/or in the joint space between two bones causes an attack. Uric acid is a natural substance resulting from the breakdown of parts of all human tissues and is found in many foods such as liver, dried beans, anchovies, and gravies. Many people with gout have excess uric acid in their blood, which may move from the blood and inflame the joints.

Treatment plans include measures to ease the pain of the attacks, prevent future attacks, stop the uric acid buildup in tissues and joint spaces, and prevent kidney stone development. Either nonsteroidal **anti-inflammatory** drugs or **corticosteroids** are usually prescribed, and patients may begin to improve within a few hours of treatment. If a patient has recurrent or frequent attacks of gout, there are different medications that may be prescribed to prevent the uric acid crystal formation.

*See also:* Chronic Disease; Genetic Disorders

**FURTHER READING**
Eustice, Carol. *Health Guide to Everything Arthritis.* Avon, Mass.: Adams Media, 2007.
Sutton, Amy, ed. *Arthritis Sourcebook.* Detroit: Omnigraphics, 2004.

# ■ ASTHMA

A lung disease in which attacks of breathlessness are caused by **chronic** airway **inflammation.** The muscles around the airways, or bronchial tubes, of the lungs can tighten up, causing the lining of the tubes to become inflamed and swollen. Once they are swollen, the airways are very sensitive and react strongly to irritants and **allergens**. As airways narrow and extra mucus is produced in the breathing passages and throat, less air flows through to the lung tissue. Breathing then becomes difficult.

### PREVALENCE

According to the National Heart Lung and Blood Institute, more than 22 million Americans have asthma. The American Lung Association

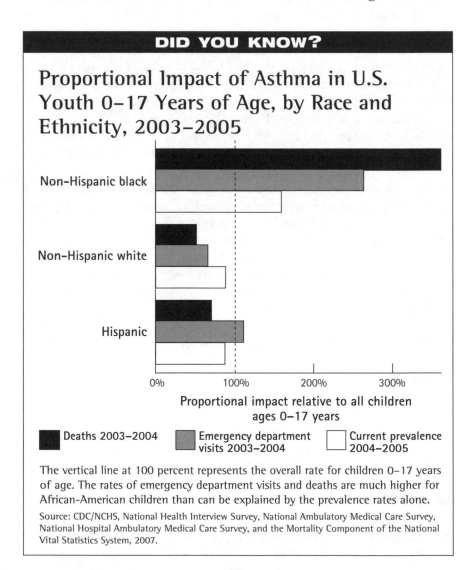

**DID YOU KNOW?**

## Proportional Impact of Asthma in U.S. Youth 0–17 Years of Age, by Race and Ethnicity, 2003–2005

Non-Hispanic black

Non-Hispanic white

Hispanic

0%          100%          200%          300%

Proportional impact relative to all children
ages 0–17 years

■ Deaths 2003–2004     ■ Emergency department     □ Current prevalence
                          visits 2003–2004            2004–2005

The vertical line at 100 percent represents the overall rate for children 0–17 years of age. The rates of emergency department visits and deaths are much higher for African-American children than can be explained by the prevalence rates alone.

Source: CDC/NCHS, National Health Interview Survey, National Ambulatory Medical Care Survey, National Hospital Ambulatory Medical Care Survey, and the Mortality Component of the National Vital Statistics System, 2007.

predicts the rate of asthma in the United States will likely double by the year 2020.

Nearly one in 10 American children has asthma, and the reason for the high incidence is not yet known. One theory for the increase is that children are spending more time indoors and are thus exposed to harmful indoor pollutants for longer periods of time.

Although asthma can start at any age, it is most common among children. About half of the cases first occur in children under the age of 10. Many children seem to outgrow all symptoms early in their teens. Although it is true that some youngsters seem to outgrow their asthma, the symptoms often return in their adult years. Still, the impact of asthma on children under the age of 17 is sometimes life-threatening.

### Heredity

Scientists theorize that heredity plays an important role in the tendency to develop asthma. In fact, **genes** linked to asthma have been discovered; and most likely the tendency is caused by a combination of genes. If one parent has asthma, there is a 40 to 50 percent chance that the child will develop the disease; if both parents have asthma, the risk increases to 80 percent or more.

Also, there appears to be a genetic-environmental role—that is, someone with the genes to develop asthma is exposed to something in the environment that causes the genes to activate, and asthma is expressed.

## TWO TYPES OF ATTACKS

Some asthma attacks can be classified as **extrinsic,** triggered by outside influences such as allergies to pollen, dust, mold spores, or animal dander (dandruff and small hairs). Other allergies to foods, drinks, drugs, paints, bleaches, household cleansers, and hair spray, perfume, or workplace chemicals can trigger attacks. A greater percentage of children (up to 85 percent) than adults (about 50 percent) suffer from extrinsic asthma. Not every asthma patient suffers from allergies.

Another type of asthma attack is **intrinsic,** triggered by exercise, sports activities, extreme weather conditions, fatigue, or stress.

## SYMPTOMS

Symptoms include coughing, wheezing (a whistling sound during breathing), tightness in the chest, and shortness of breath during attacks, which often occur at night or in the early morning. Although it is a chronic condition, symptoms are not present all the time in most patients. They appear just before and during an episode. The severity of symptoms varies greatly from person to person and in the individual asthmatic from time to time.

Symptoms range from mild to severe and can be life-threatening. However, there are usually warning signs before life-threatening asthma attacks. Usually the signs of an upcoming attack appear hours or even days before a full-blown attack develops. More serious episodes may include rapid breathing and pulse, heavy sweating, and sometimes tingling in the fingers or legs. Symptoms result in sleep disruptions and time lost from school and work. Although there is no cure for asthma, most symptoms can be controlled with appropriate treatment.

## PREVENTIVE BEHAVIORS

While there is no prevention of asthma, there are ways to prevent asthma attacks and control asthma. Most people with asthma can learn to identify the early warning signs of an asthma attack, treat the condition before it has a chance to get worse, and help to keep the asthma under control. When asthma is controlled most patients can lead an active life without symptoms, sleep through the night, and have good lung function. With regular health care and an understanding of symptoms, an asthmatic patient can often avoid an attack.

Attacks are best prevented by avoiding the allergens, irritants, and conditions that act as triggers. Asthmatics should not smoke and should avoid exposure to smoke; eliminate household cockroaches; and try to stay free of **respiratory** infections such as colds, flu, and bronchitis.

Reducing the effects of air pollution by using air conditioners and air filters, following a treatment plan, and taking medication exactly as prescribed can help prevent episodes.

## COPING AND TREATMENT

If you have asthma, you may have had some unexpected episodes of coughing, breathlessness, and/or fatigue. These episodes can be puzzling and can lead to feelings of frustration, anger, or even fear. Your asthma may affect your ability to play sports, play an instrument in the band, and sing in the choir. The good news is that you can work with your health-care provider, your parents or guardian, and your teachers and coaches to ensure you have a safe environment. Your health-care team will need to know about all the medications you take to see whether they affect your asthma. With the team, you will develop treatment goals and learn how to meet those goals.

## Asthma Guidelines

The National Asthma Education and Prevention Program (NAEPP) released updated asthma guidelines in 2007 that recommend four activities for asthma care: educating patients and their families in the management of the disease; monitoring asthma control; reducing exposure to environmental factors that worsen asthma; and taking appropriate medications.

First, the guidelines recommend that your health-care provider give you a written asthma action plan with strategies for controlling the disease both long term and short term. Part of this plan is the medication plan, designed to control symptoms.

Many patients need daily long-term control medication. The NAEPP concludes that inhaled corticosteroids, which act on the immune system to control inflammation and swelling of the bronchial tubes, will benefit most patients needing long-term control medicines. Other medications are useful for the quick relief of symptoms. You can feel the effects of these medicines within minutes.

If allergies are triggering the asthma, you may need a series of allergy shots. Allergy shots work by giving an increasingly larger dose of the allergen over time, and this gradually lessens the sensitivity to the allergen. Your health-care provider will help identify which allergens or irritants are important for you to avoid.

Regular appointments (at least every six months) with your health-care provider are important to manage asthma, as its severity may vary from season to season. At these checkups, changes in medication can be made. Additionally, this is a good time to discuss symptoms, effects of medications, and occurrences of attacks. Other parts of the checkup are a lung function test and an opportunity to ask questions and express any concerns about the treatment plan.

Asthma treatment goals include maintaining near-normal activity levels including exercise; maintaining normal or near-normal lung function test results; preventing coughing, shortness of breath, waking up at night, and lost time at school or work; preventing the need for emergency-department visits or hospitalizations; and avoiding medication side effects.

### Short-term Treatment

For short-term rescue treatment, most asthmatics will be prescribed a bronchodilator inhaler, which contains a substance that opens the bronchial tubes in a few minutes. Some call it a rescue inhaler.

Carrying the inhaler with them at all times allows asthmatics to be prepared for attacks when they are away from home. Bronchodilators widen the air passages and not only stop **acute** episodes but also prevent exercise-induced asthma. Some people prefer to use a nebulizer instead of an inhaler; it works like a vaporizer or humidifier and produces a mist that is breathed in.

The National Asthma Education and Prevention Program advises using a peak flow meter to follow the progress of an asthma attack. This inexpensive, portable device measures the airflow through the bronchial tubes and can alert you to the probability of a dangerous asthma attack.

**Long-term Treatment**

Inhaled **steroids** are the mainstay of asthmatic treatment. These medications provide an **anti-inflammatory** effect that keeps air passages open. In addition, there are several newer drugs that target the **immune response** that occurs in asthma.

Allergy shots can make asthma patients less sensitive to allergy triggers. Avoiding known triggers is also important in managing asthma.

## ASTHMA SUCCESS STORIES

Many famous people have learned to manage their asthma and have gone on to succeed: in leadership (presidents Theodore Roosevelt [1901–09], John F. Kennedy [1961–63]); in professional sports (Dennis Rodman, Emmitt Smith); and in Olympic sports (Greg Louganis, Jackie Joyner-Kersee, Nancy Hogshead). One of the 10 percent of Olympic athletes all over the world with asthma, Nancy Hogshead won four swimming medals at the 1984 Olympics. As she was about to compete for her fifth medal, an asthma attack started her on a year-long journey of discovering the warning signs of an attack and which medicines worked best for her. Nancy says of her experience, "Having asthma is no reason to be sick. It may take a while, but if you work with your doctor, you'll find the best way to treat your asthma!"

*See also:* Allergies

**FURTHER READING**

Hannaway, Paul. *The Asthma Self-Help Book.* Roddin, Calif.: Prima
   Publications, 1994.

Hogshead, Nancy, and Gerald Secor Couzens. *Asthma & Exercise.* New York: Holt, 1991.

National Heart Lung and Blood Institute. "What Is Asthma?" URL: www.nhlbi.nih.gov/health/dci/Diseases/Asthma/Asthma_WhatIs. html. Accessed July 15, 2008.

Navarra, Tova. *The Encyclopedia of Asthma and Respiratory Disorders.* New York: Facts On File, 2003.

Silverstein, Alvin, Virginia Silverstein, and Laura Silverstein Nunn. *The Asthma Update.* Berkeley Heights, N.J.: Enslow Publishers, 2006.

# ■ BIPOLAR DISORDER
*See:* Anxiety and Mood Disorders

# ■ BLOOD PRESSURE
*See:* Heart Disease

# ■ CANCER

A disease in which cells grow and multiply uncontrollably, destroying healthy tissue in the process. Cancer can sometimes result in death by crowding out normal cells, which leads to loss of tissue function. Normally, new cells are produced at the rate that other cells die. Regulating this growth are **genes**, which can mutate (change) and cause cells to divide uncontrollably.

In cancer, as the cells continue dividing, they often form **tumors**, which are abnormal tissue masses. **Malignant** tumors are cancerous and can spread the disease to tissues in other parts of the body. **Metastasis** is the process of malignant cells moving into healthy tissues, and as cells begin to metastasize, cancer is difficult to treat. Benign tumors are noncancerous and usually do not spread and cause disease.

## CAUSES

Cancer can occur in otherwise healthy people. The changes in cancer cells that regulate cell growth and division are due to **mutations** in the DNA segments that control production of proteins that regulate the cell cycle. Often, the genetic damage is repaired normally by the body, but the body's repair systems can fail, resulting in cancer.

## INCIDENCE

Cancers are rare in those under 20 years of age, but they can occur in any age group. People over age 44 are at the highest risk for developing cancer. Part of the reason for this higher risk is that a cancer can start developing in a young person and not be detected

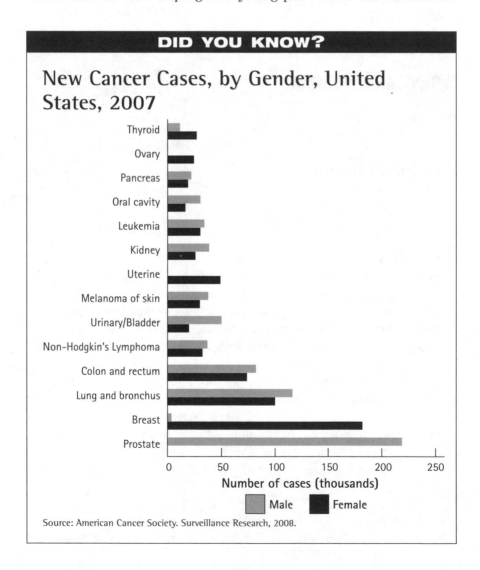

**DID YOU KNOW?**

**New Cancer Cases, by Gender, United States, 2007**

Number of cases (thousands)

■ Male   ■ Female

Source: American Cancer Society. Surveillance Research, 2008.

for many years. This makes older people seem more vulnerable even though they may have developed the disease at a much younger age. Also, older people have had more time for **genetic** mutations to do their work, and older people's **immune** systems are weaker and less able to fight back. More than one change in DNA is required to change an abnormal cell into a cancer cell. Over time, the changes in DNA accumulate. This might explain why the risk of cancer increases with age, and why cancer runs in some families. A person who inherits one or more changes from a parent is at a higher risk for developing cancer than someone who does not inherit these changes.

Environmental factors can also affect one's risk for developing cancer. Substances and agents that cause mutations in growth-controlling genes are called **carcinogens**. The three main carcinogens are chemicals, **viruses,** and radiation. Not everyone exposed to these carcinogens will get cancer, but the risk of cancer increases with exposure to them.

### PREVENTION

Avoiding carcinogens can help reduce the risk of cancer. The Food and Drug Administration (FDA) requires labels and warnings on

---

## DID YOU KNOW?

### The Most Common Teen Cancers

- Blood cells (leukemia)
- Brain and nervous system
- Immune system cells (lymphoma)
- Bones and joints
- Testicles
- Skin (melanoma)

Cancer of the bones and joints is more common among young teens, and cancers of the testicles and melanomas are more common among older teens.

Source: Surveillance Epidemiology and End Results Cancer Statistics Review, National Cancer Institute, 1975–2004.

products that might contain carcinogens. There are laws to protect people from cancer-causing chemicals, such as asbestos, in workplaces and schools. Other chemicals that increase chances of getting cancer through overexposure are benzene, coal tar, soot, formaldehyde, arsenic, nickel, and hair dyes. Most people will not be overexposed to these chemicals that can factor into cancers of the skin, lungs, blood, and bladder, because such chemicals are usually a workplace hazard in certain professions.

**Avoiding Tobacco**
Research shows that avoiding tobacco of all kinds, including secondhand smoke and smokeless tobacco, can reduce risk of cancer. Smoking is the number one risk factor for cancer; tobacco causes one-third of all cancer deaths and 90 percent of lung cancer deaths. Tobacco can also be a factor in cancers of the bladder, cervix, esophagus, larynx, and tongue.

**Diet**
A poor diet including too much fat has been linked to risks for many types of cancer. A low-fat diet that includes plenty of fruits, vegetables, legumes (beans and peas), and whole-grain products can help prevent digestive system cancers. Obesity increases the risk of cancers of the breast, ovaries, uterus, prostate, gallbladder, and pancreas. Maintaining a normal body weight is a key preventive measure

## DID YOU KNOW?

## Cigarette Smoking

Although cigarette smoking has declined significantly over the last 40 years, in 2005, there was a 1 percentage point increase in the number of high school students who smoke and a 0.4 percent increase in the number of men who smoke.

Sources: Centers for Disease Control and Prevention, National Center for Health Statistics, Data from the National Health Interview Survey, Youth Risk Behavior Survey, and the National Vital Statistics System, 2007.

**DID YOU KNOW?**

# Teen Use of Sunscreen

- 20 percent of teens never use sunscreen.
- 71 percent of teens only use sunscreen when outside for a long time.
- Only 9 percent of teens use sunscreen every day.

Despite the danger of the Sun's rays' changing skin cells into cancerous cells, most teens do not use sunscreen regularly.

Source: *Current Health 2*, April/May 2008.

against cancer. Excessive alcohol consumption increases risks of cancer of the mouth, esophagus, throat, larynx, breast, and liver.

### Radiation

Because there is a connection between the amount of ultraviolet radiation to which a person is exposed and the risk of developing skin cancer, wearing hats, staying in the shade, and using sunscreen is recommended for everyone exposed to the sun. Although sunburn is a clear sign of overexposure, you can get an overdose of solar radiation without burning, even on a cloudy day.

Because of the possible risk of leukemia and skin cancer, medical X-rays have been adjusted to emit very low doses of radiation. Wearing a lead apron during medical X-rays for dental cavities and broken bones protects against risky exposure to radiation.

### Regular Checkups

People can also increase their chances of surviving cancer by having regular medical checkups. Screening tests for cancer are very simple and are specific for the different cancer types. Some screening tests (Pap tests, mammograms, colon and rectal exams) are performed by health professionals and some tests are self-examinations (breast, skin, testicles, and lymph nodes). The earlier cancer is detected, the more likely its spread to other tissue can be halted.

## TREATMENT

Depending on the cancer type, its stage of growth, a person's age and general health, treatment plans can vary. In addition, the treatment benefit must be evaluated against its side effects, or risk.

### Methods

Drugs, surgery, and radiation are all used to treat cancer. If cancer is detected before spreading, surgery can remove the tumors. After surgery, drugs (**chemotherapy**), or radiation can help ensure all the cancer cells are destroyed. Side effects of chemotherapy have lessened in recent years due to development of new drugs. When drug therapy is used to destroy cancer cells, some normal cells are destroyed as well.

### Immunotherapy

**Immunotherapy** is a treatment approach that uses the body's own immune system to fight cancer. One of the two approaches used in immunotherapy is helping the body's immune system recognize cancer cells as foreign invaders. **Antibodies** that recognize cancer cells as foreign can be given to the person with cancer. If the person's immune system already recognizes cancer cells as foreign invaders but is not strong enough to fight them, there are injections of interferon that can be given. **Interferon** boosts the immune system's ability to fight cancer. It binds to neighboring cells and stimulates those cells to produce antiviral proteins that can prevent viruses from replicating in those cells.

### Side Effects

One side effect (usually temporary) is hair loss; another is nausea. In radiation therapy, high-energy waves from X-rays or radioactive materials are aimed at tumors, and the intense energy damages and kills cancer cells more than normal cells. Fatigue is the major side effect of radiation. Improved precision with the process is causing fewer side effects, which include **inflammation** of mucous membranes in the nose and mouth, stomach upset, and diarrhea.

### Treatment Success Rates

The rates of successfully treating cancers are rising as researchers amass more and more data about prevention and treatment. One study shows that more than 10 million Americans now living have had cancer, with three-fourths of them now living cancer-free. Still, cancer remains the second-leading cause of death after coronary heart disease in the United States.

## TYPES OF CANCER

There are many types of cancer, but some of the most common types include breast cancer, cervical cancer, colon cancer, ovarian cancer, prostate cancer, and skin cancer. Each type is screened for differently, each affects certain groups more than others, and treatment varies for each.

### Breast Cancer

Breast cancer affects one in eight women in their lifetime. However, the risk is higher the longer a woman lives. It is the second most common cause of cancer death in women and the main cause of death in women ages 45–55.

Risk factors for breast cancer are many. The first is age—the older one is, the higher the risk. Most cases occur in women over age 60. A personal history of breast cancer raises the risk of a subsequent cancer. If a woman has a mother, sister, or daughter with breast cancer, the risk is higher, especially if the relative got breast cancer before age 40. Having other relatives with breast cancer on the mother's side is a possible risk factor. Having abnormal cells from the breast also presents a risk factor. Recently, a screening method to obtain cell samples has been developed, although it is not yet widely used.

Gene changes run in certain families. Those at high risk due to their ethnicity or family history may decide to undergo gene testing. But gene testing is not to be done lightly, as it has many implications. Some people can face future refusals for coverage if insurance companies discover the person has high-risk genes. The other issue is what to do with the information if the gene tests come back positive. Some women can choose just to be vigilant about breast self-exams and keeping up to date on their physical exams and mammograms. Some choose breast removal before breast cancer can develop. The psychological implications vary widely in the women who choose this. Some feel glad that they have made a proactive choice to live longer, and some are profoundly affected by the loss of their breasts. The other issue is whether having this information and worrying is better than not having it. Therefore, before any type of gene testing, a genetics counselor must sit down and lay out the whole picture of what the person is getting into.

Exposure to hormones—whether one's own or synthetic—have an impact on a woman's risk of breast cancer. The older a woman is when she has her first child, the higher the risk. Women who do not have children have a higher risk also. Women who start menstruating before age 12 and go through menopause after age 55 have a higher risk, presumably from a longer period of exposure to estrogen. Studies have shown that women who take estrogen plus progestin as hormone replacement therapy have a higher risk of breast cancer, especially the longer they have taken this combination. However, there is *no* relationship between abortion or miscarriage and breast cancer.

Race is a factor in breast cancer risk. White women have a higher incidence of breast cancer, but African-American women tend to be diagnosed later and with more aggressive types of breast cancer.

A history of radiation therapy to the chest before age 30 increases the risk for breast cancer. Women who have denser breasts on mammograms have higher risks of breast cancer. Women who took DES (a synthetic hormone) between 1940 and 1971 are at higher risk. Their daughters are being evaluated to determine if they also have a higher risk.

Being overweight or obese after menopause is a risk factor for breast cancer. Estrogen is stored in the fat cells and thus overweight and obese women have more estrogen exposure. Women who have been physically inactive through their lives are at an increased risk of breast cancer. Studies also show that the more alcohol a woman drinks, the greater her risk of breast cancer.

Prevention begins with avoiding smoking and maintaining a healthy weight and remaining active through one's life. Reducing a woman's alcohol intake reduces her risk of breast cancer. Some women with precancerous cell changes may elect to take hormonal medicines to block female hormones.

Early detection is now possible with mammograms. Mammograms are a special type of X-ray that views the breast tissue and structures. Its goal is to look for tumors, calcium deposits that might indicate cancer, and other changes associated with cancer. The National Cancer Institute recommends screening mammograms after age 40 every one to two years. If a woman is at higher risk, she should discuss with her health-care provider beginning mammograms or other screening exams earlier. A clinical breast exam (an exam done by a health-care provider) on a regular basis also is important and recommended. Breast self-exams (BSE) have not been shown to reduce death rates from breast cancer, but many health-care providers and organizations continue to recommend them to patients, feeling that a patient may detect a change between physical exams.

After a suspicious lump or area is found, a **biopsy** will usually be done. In a biopsy, a needle is usually inserted into the area, and specimens are sent away to the lab for evaluation under the microscope. If a biopsy is positive, it means that cancerous cells were found and the patient is diagnosed with cancer. Often a patient will seek a second opinion in deciding treatment.

Treatments include different types of surgery, from a lumpectomy to take out only the bad area to removal of the breast and underlying muscles and lymph nodes up to the arm. The stage at which the cancer is found usually guides the treatment. Sometimes surgery may be all that is necessary to treat a small and well-defined cancer, but usually chemotherapy is prescribed to kill any remaining cancer cells. Some patients have chemotherapy first to shrink a large tumor. Radiation is also often used. The radiation beams also kill any remaining cancer cells.

Select patients receive hormone therapy. Women get tested to see if they have a type of cancer that needs hormones to grow. If so, then the doctors prescribe other types of hormones to block the female's own estrogen so any remaining cancer cells cannot grow.

Newer biological therapy is being used if breast cancer has spread. These drugs help the body's immune system fight if the patient is shown to have too much of a certain protein. The side effects can be severe and include heart damage.

### Cervical Cancer

The cervix is the opening to the uterus. Cervical cancer is classified by the microscopic evaluation of a tissue sample obtained on a Pap smear. Cervical cancers start with a precancerous change and over time, if untreated, will progress to cancer. Usually considered a slow-growing cancer that takes years to emerge, it can occur in under a year. Treating precancerous changes will prevent cancer in most women. The key to cervical cancer prevention and treatment is early detection.

The most important risk factor is the HPV (human papillomavirus) infection. There are 100 types of HPV, but only a few high-risk types. Two-thirds of all cervical cancers are caused by HPV-16 and HPV-18. HPV is spread in skin to skin contact including vaginal, anal, and oral sex.

Women should undergo a yearly pelvic and Pap test. The pelvic exam involves the health-care provider inserting a speculum into the woman's vaginal opening and looking at the opening to the uterus—the cervix—taking a sample of tissue from different parts of the cervix, and palpating the woman's ovaries. The Pap test is the taking of fluid for microscopic evaluation in a laboratory. The Pap looks at the cervical cells for changes caused by HPV. Some health-care providers use the HPV test as well.

If the tests find a high risk HPV or certain changes associated with precancerous or cancerous cervical changes, then a colposcopy procedure will be done. A colposcopy is similar to a pelvic exam and its insertion of the speculum, but the health-care provider has a special binocular lens so he or she can see the abnormalities clearly and can apply acetic acid to the abnormal areas. Further treatments can include taking out tissue as necessary or applying cryosurgery (destruction or removal of tissue by freezing). An advanced case of cervical cancer may mean the entire uterus and cervix would need to be removed, but this is rare with the institution of regular Pap screenings.

Prevention of cervical cancer has been a subject of much discussion due to the identification of the HPV varieties associated highly with this cancer. The release and recommendation of use of the HPV vaccine has received a lot of media attention. For this vaccine to be useful, it must be administered before a girl becomes sexually active. Many parents are uncomfortable with the idea that they are giving "permission" to their daughter to engage in sexual intercourse, while other parents welcome a chance for their daughter to avoid the risk of cervical cancer.

Several other measures are helpful in prevention of cervical cancer. Condoms are helpful but do not offer complete protection. Smoking appears to make the cervix vulnerable, so not smoking is an important measure to take. Prevention of other sexually transmitted diseases, such as HIV and chlamydia, reduces the chances of cervical cancer. Chlamydia is associated with a higher cervical cancer risk, and HIV can hurt the body's ability to fight an HPV infection. A diet high in fruits and vegetables is recommended. Having multiple pregnancies or taking oral contraceptives for many years also increases the risk of cervical cancer.

Other risk factors for cervical cancer include low socioeconomic status and having a family history of cervical cancer in a mother or sister. Women whose mothers took DES when pregnant with them also face increased risk of cervical cancer.

## Colon and Rectal Cancer

Colorectal cancer is cancer that starts in the colon or rectum. The colon, or large intestine, is about five feet long, and the last six inches are the rectum, where waste leaves the body.

Most colon cancers grow slowly over several years and begin as a polyp—tissue overgrowth from the colon lining that may or may not be cancer. Removing polyps virtually eliminates colon cancer.

Colon cancer is the third most common cancer in men and women. Colorectal cancer caused almost 50,000 deaths in 2008. However, the death rate has been declining for 15 years. More people are getting screened and having polyps removed before they become cancerous. Treatments are also improving for colorectal cancer.

Most colon cancer cases (90 percent) are diagnosed in people over age 50. A history of polyps or colorectal cancer will increase one's risk of developing it again. Individuals who have certain bowel diseases called Crohn's disease or ulcerative colitis have a higher risk of colon cancer because these diseases leave the colon lining inflamed for long periods of time. Family history of colorectal cancer can be a risk factor, especially if a family member had colorectal cancer under age 60. Some families have a type of syndrome where family members get large numbers of polyps and have an increased risk of a polyp becoming cancerous. African Americans and Ashkenazi Jews have a higher risk, although it is not known why.

Additionally certain lifestyle characteristics may raise one's risk of colon cancer. A diet high in red meats or cooking meats at high temperatures raises the risk. People who lack exercise, are overweight, or smoke have a higher risk of colon cancer. People who drink alcohol have a higher risk of colon cancer and those with diabetes also have an increased risk.

Prevention of colon cancer is key. Regular colon screening can virtually prevent colon cancer. Eating a diet high in fruits, vegetables, and whole grains while limiting high-fat foods is important. Research studies recommend exercise for 30 minutes, five days a week. Emerging evidence on the importance of calcium, vitamin D, and a multivitamin containing folic acid or folate encourages the use of these supplements, but further research is needed to confirm these results. Aspirin and other nonsteroidal anti-inflammatory drugs, including COX-2 inhibitors such as Celebrex, have been shown to reduce polyps for some people and may be very useful in high-risk families or individuals. This decision needs to be made with the health-care provider due to an increased risk of bleeding disorders. While hormone replacement therapy has been shown to reduce the risk of colon cancer, those on HRT who do get colon cancer often get a fast-growing type. The health-care provider should help evaluate this and other risks of hormone replacement therapy.

The flexible sigmoidoscopy is a test in which a patient cleans out his or her colon and the doctor inserts a tube with a light on it up through the rectum into about two feet of the five-foot colon to look for polyps or any abnormalities on the colon lining. The colonoscopy is similar to the sigmoidoscopy, but the patient is sedated and the tube goes the entire length of the colon. With the colonoscopy, the doctor can view the colon, but can also remove any polyp or suspect area or take a biopsy of tissue. A double contrast barium enema involves a chalky paste used to partly fill and open up the colon while air is pumped in, allowing good X-rays to be taken. This is an older and less expensive method than sigmoidoscopy or colonoscopy.

Virtual colonoscopy involves a similar type of clean-out as the sigmoidoscopy and colonoscopy, but it is not invasive. This method uses images from a CT scan or MRI to create a three-dimensional view of the large intestine. Some organizations have not wholeheartedly endorsed it, wondering if the views of the colon are satisfactory. Additionally, if something is found, the preparation has to be redone and the patient has to undergo colonoscopy. Insurance for this is not common.

A very cheap test that can be done at home is a fecal blood test, whereby a patient collects some stool at home, applies it to a special card, and returns to the medical office. The office can then test for hidden blood. Some people are put off by this test and do not follow through with it. One concern is that before bleeding occurs and can be detected, a cancer can grow to a later stage where it is harder to treat.

Early colon cancer often has no symptoms. Symptoms that may occur are a change in bowel habits such as diarrhea, constipation, or a narrowed stool for more than a few days. The person may notice feeling the need to have a bowel movement that does not go away even after having a bowel movement. Of concern is rectal bleeding, dark stools, blood in the stool, cramping or abdominal pain, and weakness and tiredness.

The treatment for colorectal cancer usually involves surgery to take out the affected area, and the remaining parts of the colon are usually sewn together. Sometimes a patient may have to have an opening called a colostomy where the stool goes into a bag from a hole going through the abdominal wall to the colon. Currently, most surgeons try to sew up the areas during the initial surgery or after a period of healing. Some patients, however, are left with a colostomy bag. Radiation therapy is often used with either external radiation beams or the insertion of radiation pellets in or around the cancer. Chemotherapy can also treat colorectal cancer.

Early diagnosis of colorectal cancer gives very successful survival rates, but if diagnosed in stage IV (the last stage) only 8 percent survive.

## Ovarian Cancer

Ovarian cancer begins in the ovaries, the part of the woman's reproductive system where eggs originate. Ovarian cancer is usually categorized by what type of cell overgrowth causes the tumor to originate. Ovarian cancer is the eighth most common cancer in women. Over 15,000 women died in 2008 from ovarian cancer. Two-thirds are age 55 or older, and ovarian cancer occurs more commonly in white women than in African-American women.

Although many theories abound, researchers do not know what causes ovarian cancer, but they do have risk factors identified. As with most cancers, the more advanced one's age, the higher the risk. It is more common after menopause, and over half of patients are over age 63 at diagnosis. Overweight and obese women face increased risk. Women who have not had children, been pregnant, or breastfed have a higher risk, and researchers believe this is related to the lifetime exposure to estrogen. Likewise, using the fertility drug Clomid (clomiphene) for more than a year, especially if no pregnancy results, or taking estrogen replacement after menopause increases the risk. Taking a synthetic male hormone called danazol increases the risk. A family history of ovarian, breast, or colorectal cancer increases the risk of ovarian cancer, as does the history of breast cancer in the woman herself. The use of talcum powder on the genital area is believed to increase the risk although since 1973 talc products must be free of asbestos; whether there is difference with newer products is not yet known. Smoking and a diet high in fat also increase the risk of ovarian cancer.

Prevention recommendations are few and should always be implemented only after serious discussion with one's health-care provider. The use of oral contraceptives over five years and having a tubal ligation or hysterectomy reduces the risk of ovarian cancer.

Ovarian cancer is difficult to find, and this is one reason for the history of poor outcomes. An annual pelvic exam by a health-care provider is recommended, but a tumor must be of a certain size to be felt and, if a woman is overweight or obese, the mass can be even more difficult to feel on exam. Symptoms are vague and can be related to many conditions. Some of the symptoms are the following: abdominal bloating, pelvic pressure, or stomach pain; trouble eating or feeling full quickly; a need to urinate often or a sense of needing to urinate urgently; tiredness; nausea; back pain; pain during sex; constipation; and menstrual changes. If an abnormality is suspected, the health-care provider usually orders an ultrasound, although many other tests, such as CT scans, may follow.

The treatment for ovarian cancer usually includes surgical removal, chemotherapy, and radiation. As with most cancers, the earlier the detection, the better the outcome. The lack of an early, accessible screening test is a major barrier to preventing deaths from ovarian cancer.

### Prostate Cancer

The prostate is a gland in the male below the bladder and above the rectum whose job is to produce fluid and aid sperm fertility. Often with aging, especially beyond age 50, the prostate will enlarge, but this enlargement is usually benign (not cancerous). The median age at diagnosis is 68 years. There are 156.7 white men per 100,000 diagnosed and 248.5 African-American men per 100,000 diagnosed with prostate cancer. The reasons for this have not been clearly identified.

Prostate cancer is the most common cancer affecting men except for skin cancer. One of the reasons it is increasingly detected is the development of a simple screening test—the PSA, or prostate specific antigen. The normal PSA level is less than 4.0, and when there are elevations or a big jump in the number (say from .25 to 3.1 in one year) the health-care provider becomes concerned about prostate cancer and orders further testing.

The physical exam may reveal an abnormality on the prostate—a hard lump—but a physical exam cannot access the entire prostate, so this alone does not provide a reliable screening method. Once an abnormal PSA or exam raises suspicions, the standard for diagnosis is a prostate biopsy, in which the doctor takes a sample of tissue from various parts of the prostate.

Most patients are diagnosed with no symptoms, although some may have urinary symptoms—feeling the need to urinate immediately, needing to urinate at night, going often to urinate, or difficulty urinating.

Once a diagnosis is established, the patient and urologist (a doctor specializing in diseases of the urinary system, including the prostate) must decide on the treatment course. Because prostate cancer can grow very slowly, some older men choose to simply watch things. In fact this common practice has raised the issue of whether screening should be performed in the population over age 75. The theory is that screening only makes the patient worry about a disease he is not going to treat and that may well not even cause his death. Others argue that the patient should know and have the option to pursue treatment or not.

Treatment choices vary widely for prostate cancer. As indicated above, many choose only to monitor the PSA levels and follow symptoms. Surgery is a common treatment, and the approaches to the surgery also vary. One approach to the surgery is to try to make it as minimally invasive as possible, which reduces complications. Other types of surgery can result in quite a bit of tissue removal. Complications of surgery can include incontinence (loss of control of the bladder) and impotence (inability to have sexual intercourse), so the decision about what type of treatment to pursue has many implications. Radiation therapy applies external radiation to the prostate, but it also has potential for complications. Cryosurgery, which involves freezing cancerous areas on the prostate, is another treatment option. Hormones to block the male hormones, or androgens, are another treatment choice. In recent years, chemotherapy has become increasingly used for prostate cancer as well.

Although study results have been mixed, the American Cancer Society recommends eating a diet rich in fruits and vegetables, especially foods high in lycopenes, a substance which may prevent DNA damage and prevent prostate cancer. The goal is five or more fruits and vegetables per day. Selenium, a mineral available as a supplement, may help lower prostate cancer risk. The drug finasteride (Proscar) reduced the risk of getting cancer by 25 percent, but those who did get prostate cancer had more aggressive types, and the side effects of the medication were significant.

## Skin Cancer

Skin cancer forms in the tissues of the skin. There are three main types of skin cancer. The most dangerous type is melanoma; the other two, basal cell carcinoma and squamous cell cancer, are considered the non-melanoma types.

Basal cell carcinoma is the most common type. It forms in the basal cells, which are in the lower part of the epidermis, the outermost layer of skin. It is most commonly found body areas exposed to the Sun, such as the head and neck.

Squamous cell skin cancer starts on the upper part of the epidermis. It usually occurs on Sun-exposed areas and commonly affects the face, ears, neck, lips, and back of the hands. It presents slightly more danger of spreading to other tissues than basal cell carcinoma, but it is not common for this to spread.

Basal and squamous cell skin cancers present the same risk factors. UV radiation from the Sun itself or from tanning lamps presents the biggest threat. Living in a sunny place year-round gives one a higher risk simply due to the time of exposure to the Sun. Likewise, the older one is, the higher the risk is due to a longer time of Sun exposure.

Men have twice the rate of basal cell and three times the rate of squamous cell cancers. Fair-skinned individuals have less melanin in the skin and are at higher risk for these skin cancers. Exposure to large amounts of arsenic, a common ingredient in insecticide, increases the risk of skin cancer. Therefore, a fair-haired male who works during the summer doing lawn care and applying insecticide to lawns would be at higher risk than a darker skinned woman working in an office. Additional risk factors include a history of radiation treatment, a history of skin cancer or skin damage from other diseases or scars, a weak immune system, HPV infection, smoking (which increases risk in squamous cell but not basal cell cancer), and genetics. Psoriasis patients who have had UV light treatment also have an increased risk.

Prevention efforts aim to reduce UV exposure. Limit sunlight exposure and protect yourself when outside. The American Cancer Society is trying to simplify the message with the marketing campaign "Slip, Slop, Slap, and Wrap": Slip on a shirt, slop on sunscreen, slap on a hat, and wrap on sunglasses. Sunscreen should have an SPF (sun protection factor) of 15 or higher, and it should be reapplied every two hours and after swimming and sweating.

Treatment of non-melanoma skin cancers is usually limited to removal by minor surgery of one type or another. If the cancer is deeper or has spread, the treatment becomes more intense. A topical medication may be used at times instead of or in addition to minor surgery. Cryosurgery (freezing of tissue) may be done as well.

Melanocyte cells are deeper in the skin, and at this level melanoma can form. Melanoma is a very serious type of cancer because it can easily spread to the lymph system. Surgical treatment usually requires fairly deep and wide incisions to get rid of all the affected areas.

Melanoma most often starts on the trunk, or midsection, of fair-skinned men and lower legs of fair-skinned women, but it can start in other areas. It is curable in early forms, but it is likely to spread to other parts of the body if not found early. If it spreads, it becomes a serious cancer very quickly. Melanoma makes up only 5 percent of skin cancers but is the most serious, claiming more than 8,000 lives each year.

The cause of melanoma is not known but risk factors have been identified. UV light exposure is the biggest risk factor, whether from sunlight or tanning beds. Patients who have large numbers of moles are known to have a higher risk of developing melanoma and should get regular skin exams and do their own self-exams monthly. Fair-skinned people, especially those with red or blond hair and freckles, have a higher risk of melanoma. If one has had a family member with melanoma or has personally had melanoma in the past, that person's risk is higher. Melanoma can occur in younger people, but it is more common in older people. Men's risk is higher than women's for developing melanoma.

Prevention of melanoma begins with the "Slip, Slap, Slop, and Wrap" program from the American Cancer Society. Children should be carefully protected from sunburn because childhood burns have been related to melanoma; additionally it teaches skin-care lessons the child can apply throughout life. Tanning beds must be avoided; there is growing research associating them with melanoma. One theory is that the UV rays in tanning beds go deeper into the skin—where the melanocytes lie. Any abnormal moles should be checked by a health-care professional and removed.

Everyone should learn the ABCDEs of melanoma. Asymmetry means one side of a mole is different from the other side. Border irregularity means the edges of the mole are ragged and blurred—not easily defined. Color means the mole has different shades of color. Diameter means the mole is larger than 6mm, ¼ inch, or the size of a pencil eraser. Evolving means a mole that is changing and growing, which should be evaluated by a dermatologist—a doctor specializing in skin diseases. If the doctor thinks you have a skin cancer, he or she will do a skin biopsy where a sample of the area is removed and examined under a microscope.

If the doctor thinks the cancer has spread to the lymph glands, he or she will do a sentinel lymph node biopsy. A radioactive liquid and blue dye are injected into the melanoma area and the lymph nodes are checked for radioactivity. If it shows up in lymph nodes, the nodes need surgical removal.

Surgery is the main treatment for most melanomas. Surgical removal may cure early melanoma. Lymph nodes that have tested positive for activity may be removed. Right now it is uncertain how helpful this is in saving lives.

Chemotherapy is used to treat melanoma that has spread from the site. Immunotherapy, which is therapy to boost the patient's immune system, is used in advanced melanoma, although the side effects can be harsh. Radiation therapy may be used to shrink the cancer.

Researchers are working on **vaccines** that may be a possibility for preventive help in the future.

*See also:* Chronic Disease; Genetic Disorders; Leukemia; Skin Disorders; Treatment

**FURTHER READING**
Anderson, John, and Larry Trivieri, eds. *Alternative Medicine: The Definitive Guide.* Berkeley, Calif.: Celestial Arts, 2002.
Teeley, Peter, and Philip Bashe. *The Complete Cancer Survival Guide.* New York: Broadway, 2005.

# ■ CARDIOVASCULAR DISEASE
*See:* Heart Disease

# ■ CATARACTS
*See:* Eye Disorders

# ■ CENTERS FOR DISEASE CONTROL AND PREVENTION (CDC)
A part of the U.S. Department of Health and Human Services, which is the primary federal agency for conducting and supporting public health activities in the United States. The CDC promotes health protection through awareness, prevention, and preparedness. The CDC focuses on occupational safety and health, environmental health and injury prevention, health information services, health promotion, **infectious** diseases, global health, terrorism preparedness, and emergency response.

## GOALS
One of the goals of the CDC is to help all people, including those at greatest risk of illness, to live their optimal life span with the highest quality of health in every stage of life. This includes increasing the number of infants and children who have a strong start for healthy and safe lives, increasing the number of adolescents who are prepared to be

## DID YOU KNOW?

# The Mission of the CDC

The mission of the CDC is to promote health and quality of life by preventing and controlling disease, injury, and disability. The CDC seeks to accomplish its mission by working with partners throughout the nation and the world to:

- Monitor health
- Detect and investigate health problems
- Conduct research to enhance prevention
- Develop and advocate sound public health policies
- Implement prevention strategies
- Promote healthy behaviors
- Foster safe and healthful environments
- Provide leadership and training

Source: Centers for Disease Control and Prevention, 2007.

healthy, productive, independent members of society, and increasing the number of adults who are able to fully participate in life activities as they live longer, enjoying high-quality, productive, independent lives.

A second goal is to ensure that people live, work, learn, and play in healthy environments. This includes reducing the numbers of workplace illnesses, injuries, and fatalities; promoting healthy lunches and physical education programs in schools; increasing the health, safety, and equitable distribution of health care; and preventing illness and injury during travel and recreation. Another goal is preventing public health disasters by protecting people against infectious, occupational, environmental, and terrorist threats. Another goal is to be a resource for global health promotion, protection, and diplomacy. This includes improving global health through medical technology, international coalitions, government interventions, and promotion of basic behavior changes.

The CDC gathers data on diseases, helps determine the causes of epidemics and other health problems, and promotes ways to prevent diseases. It provides the latest information on diseases to consumers, scientists, and government officials.

*See also:* AIDS; Arthritis; Asthma; Cancer; Chicken Pox; Chronic Disease; Genetic Disorders; Diabetes Mellitus (DM); Epidemics and Pandemics; Heart Disease; Hepatitis; Immunization; Influenza; Leukemia; Lyme Disease; Measles; Mononucleosis, Infectious; Multiple Sclerosis; Parkinson's Disease; Sexually Transmitted Diseases (STDs); Skin Disorders; Treatment

**FURTHER READING**

Centers for Disease Control and Prevention. "About the CDC." URL: http://www.cdc.gov/about.

# ■ CEREBRAL PALSY

A group of disorders resulting from injury to parts of the brain or from a problem with development that affects a person's ability to move and keep balance and posture. *Cerebral* refers to the brain; *palsy* refers to weakness or problems using muscles. The developmental problem often happens before, during, or soon after birth.

**Genetic** conditions and problems with blood supply to the brain can affect how a child's brain develops during the first six months of pregnancy. After the brain has developed, causes of cerebral palsy can include bacterial meningitis and other **infections**, bleeding in the brain, lack of oxygen, severe jaundice, and head injury.

The degree of disability from the disease can range from a little clumsiness and awkwardness to the inability to walk. Cerebral palsy is the most common cause of motor disability in childhood. It affects one in 278 children in the United States. The part of the brain that is damaged determines what parts of the body are affected.

## SYMPTOMS

Because there are many different types and levels of disability, the symptoms of cerebral palsy vary greatly. A major sign of the disorder is a delay in reaching the motor or movement milestones for a child's age. For example, children more than two months old with cerebral palsy might have difficulty in controlling their heads when picked up and have stiff legs that cross when they are picked up. Other examples are children unable to crawl at 12 months or walk at 24 months.

## Q & A

**Question: Why do the disabilities of children with cerebral palsy differ so much from one child to another?**

**Answer:** Cerebral palsy causes different types of weaknesses and problems in each child. Problems in different parts of the brain cause problems in different parts of the body.

### PREVENTIVE BEHAVIORS AND TREATMENT

Some head injuries that cause cerebral palsy are preventable with car seats and sports helmets. The type of cerebral palsy caused by jaundice can be prevented by using special lights (phototherapy) shortly after an infant is born. Although cerebral palsy cannot be cured, treatment can help a person take as active a part as possible in family, school, and social life. Treatments can include physical and occupational therapy, medicine, operations, and leg braces.

*See also:* Chronic Disease; Treatment

#### FURTHER READING

Bjorklund, Ruth. *Cerebral Palsy.* Tarrytown, N.Y.: Marshall Cavendish, 2007.
Shannon, Joyce Brennfleck, ed. *Movement Disorders Sourcebook.* Detroit: Omnigraphics, 2003.

## ■ CHICKEN POX

A highly **contagious** viral disease that is usually mild but can be serious, even in healthy children. A **vaccine** for chicken pox became available in the United States in 1995. Before that, about 4 million people, mostly children, contracted the disease each year. Caused by the varicella-zoster **virus,** which is part of a group of viruses called herpesviruses, chicken pox spreads easily through the air and by physical contact. The chicken pox vaccine is a safe, effective way to prevent chicken pox and its possible complications. In the small number of cases in which the vaccine doesn't stop chicken pox completely, the resulting **infection** is mild.

# Q & A

## Question: What are the risks of the chicken pox vaccine?

**Answer:** Although the risk of the chicken pox vaccine causing serious illness or death is very small, the vaccine could cause serious problems in those who are allergic to it. Most people who get the chicken pox vaccine have no problems, but reactions are more likely after the first dose than after the second. One out of five children experience soreness or swelling at the site of the shot; one out of 10 get a fever; one out of 25 get a mild rash up to a month following vaccination. Very rarely do seizures and pneumonia result from the chicken pox vaccine.

## SYMPTOMS

The major symptom is a red, itchy rash that breaks out on the face, scalp, chest, and back, but it can spread across the entire body, even into the throat, eyes, and vagina. The rash usually appears less than two weeks after exposure to the virus. Starting out as superficial spots, the blisters quickly fill with liquid, break open, and crust over. For several days, the spots continue to appear, and the itching can be intense. Other symptoms that often occur with the rash are fever, headache, abdominal pain, loss of appetite, discomfort, irritability, mild cough, and runny nose.

## RISK FACTORS

Anyone who has not been vaccinated or who has never had the disease is at risk of contracting chicken pox. A person who has the disease can transmit the virus for up to 48 hours before the rash appears and until all the spots crust over. The disease can spread quickly within child-care facilities, schools, and families. Direct contact with the rash or droplets dispersed into the air by coughing or sneezing spreads the disease.

## COMPLICATIONS

Although chicken pox is normally a mild childhood disease, it can become serious and lead to complications for high-risk groups such as teens, adults, pregnant women, and newborns and infants whose mothers never had chicken pox or the vaccine. People taking **steroid** medications, those with eczema, and those with impaired **immune systems** are also at risk of complications. A bacterial skin infection is the most common complication. Very serious complications are pneumonia and encephalitis, an **inflammation** of the brain.

## SHINGLES

Shingles is a painful band of short-lived blisters that reactivate many years later from the varicella-zoster viruses that have remained in some nerve cells. The blisters, which can be extremely painful, appear along the nerve pathways. Although the shingles can last for up to five weeks, after the rash has healed discomfort along the nerve pathways can last months or even years. Fever, chills, and sensitivity along the nerve pathways are early symptoms. Then a rash of red spots appears, followed by blisters filled with the virus. Older adults and people with weakened immune systems are likely to be the one in 10 adults who experience shingles years after having chicken pox.

## TREATMENT AND PREVENTION

Simple self-care measures to take once chicken pox is contracted are not scratching (which can cause scarring), taking cool baths and applying lotion to relieve itching, getting lots of rest, eating a bland diet, and treating a fever—but not with aspirin, due to the risk of contracting Reye's syndrome. No medical treatment is required for normally healthy children with chicken pox. A health-care provider may prescribe an **antihistamine** for relief of itching. If someone falls into a high-risk group, an antiviral drug may lessen the disease's severity. In some cases, the vaccine taken after exposure to the virus can prevent or lessen the severity of the disease.

### Reye's Syndrome

No child or adult with chicken pox should take any medicine containing aspirin because the combination of chicken pox and aspirin has been associated with Reye's syndrome. Reye's syndrome is an illness causing brain inflammation and fat buildup in the liver. The symptoms start with nausea and vomiting and progress to confusion, agitation, seizures, and coma. About 20 children per year get Reye's syndrome, and most recover, although it can be deadly.

### Prevention

The best prevention is the chicken pox vaccine, which provides complete protection from the virus for nearly 90 percent of the children receiving it. The vaccine is not approved for pregnant women, people with weakened immunity, and people allergic to gelatin or the **antibiotic** neomycin.

*See also:* Immunizations; Infections, Bacterial and Viral; Treatment

**FURTHER READING**

Plum, Jennifer. *Everything You Need to Know about Chicken Pox and Shingles*. New York: Rosen, 2001.

## ■ CHRONIC DISEASE

An illness that lasts a long time, is generally noninfectious in origin, and is unlikely to be curable. Examples are diabetes, hypertension, and heart disease.

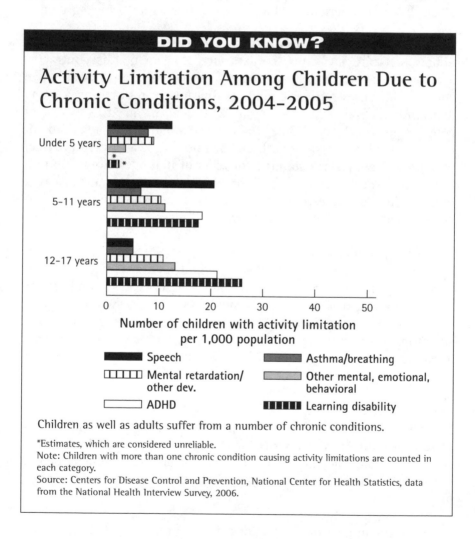

**DID YOU KNOW?**

**Activity Limitation Among Children Due to Chronic Conditions, 2004–2005**

Number of children with activity limitation per 1,000 population

Legend:
- Speech
- Asthma/breathing
- Mental retardation/other dev.
- Other mental, emotional, behavioral
- ADHD
- Learning disability

Children as well as adults suffer from a number of chronic conditions.

*Estimates, which are considered unreliable.
Note: Children with more than one chronic condition causing activity limitations are counted in each category.
Source: Centers for Disease Control and Prevention, National Center for Health Statistics, data from the National Health Interview Survey, 2006.

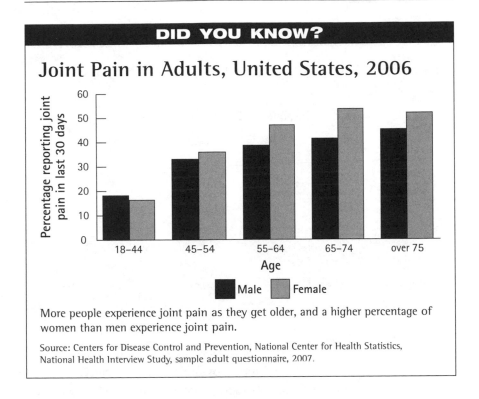

**DID YOU KNOW?**

## Joint Pain in Adults, United States, 2006

More people experience joint pain as they get older, and a higher percentage of women than men experience joint pain.

Source: Centers for Disease Control and Prevention, National Center for Health Statistics, National Health Interview Study, sample adult questionnaire, 2007.

## PREVALENCE

During the last century, the nature of diseases causing the most death, illness, and disability among Americans has changed dramatically. Costly and preventable **chronic** diseases kill seven of every 10 Americans who die each year, or more than 1.7 million people. The prolonged length and disabling effects of chronic diseases result in pain, suffering, and decreased quality of life for millions of Americans. As of 2005, more than one of every 10 Americans, or 25 million people, had major limitations in their activities due to chronic diseases.

## COSTS

The medical care costs of people with chronic diseases account for more than 75 percent of the nation's $2 trillion of health-care spending. A positive trend in chronic disease is the decline in cancer and cancer deaths in recent years, yet cancer still costs the nation an estimated $89 billion annually. Although there has been a decline in the number of children using tobacco since the late 1980s and 1990s, there has been

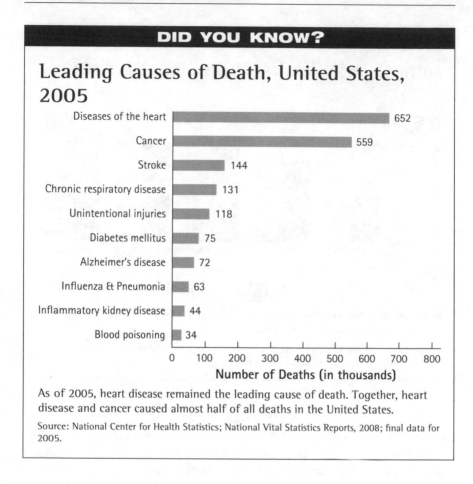

**DID YOU KNOW?**

# Leading Causes of Death, United States, 2005

As of 2005, heart disease remained the leading cause of death. Together, heart disease and cancer caused almost half of all deaths in the United States.

Source: National Center for Health Statistics; National Vital Statistics Reports, 2008; final data for 2005.

less success in lowering the rate of adults using tobacco. Costs associated with smoking exceed $193 billion annually. There is an increase in the number of diabetes cases, resulting in direct and indirect costs of diabetes being $174 billion per year. Obesity is probably the main factor behind negative trends in chronic diseases. The estimated total cost of obesity was nearly $117 billion in 2000.

## PREVENTIVE BEHAVIORS

Treating chronic disease can be difficult and expensive. Primary prevention strategies are avoiding tobacco and excessive alcohol consumption, eating a low-fat, vegetable-rich diet, avoiding excess body weight, and exercising regularly. Secondary prevention strategies are detecting the presence of diseases before symptoms occur. Early detection allows for early and more effective treatment.

*See also:* Allergies; Arthritis; Cancer; Diabetes Mellitus (DM); Centers for Disease Control and Prevention (CDC); Treatment

**FURTHER READING**

Becker, Gretchen. *The First Year—Type 2 Diabetes.* New York: Marlowe, 2007.

Lipsky, Martin, and Marla Mendelson. *The American Medical Association Guide to Preventing and Treating Heart Disease: Essential Information.* Hoboken, N.J.: Wiley, 2008.

# ■ CHRONIC OBSTRUCTIVE PULMONARY DISEASE (COPD)

A progressive illness that permanently damages the lungs and is usually caused by smoking. COPD is comprised of two illnesses, emphysema and chronic bronchitis, and kills 120,000 Americans per year; it is the fourth leading cause of death. It is expected to be the third leading cause of death by the year 2020, according to the Centers for Disease Control and Prevention.

At least 12 million Americans are known to have COPD, and studies suggest that about 12 million more cases have not been diagnosed. More than half the patients are under 65, and the disease has left about 900,000 working-age people too sick to work. COPD often goes undiagnosed, or is misdiagnosed as asthma, and left untreated.

*See also:* Chronic Diseases

**FURTHER READING**

Shimberg, Elaine Fantle. *Coping with COPD: Understanding, Treating, and Living with Chronic Obstructive Pulmonary Disease.* New York: St. Martin's Griffin, 2003.

# ■ CONJUNCTIVITIS

*See:* Eye Disorders

# ■ CYSTIC FIBROSIS

*See:* Genetic Disorders

# ■ DEMENTIA
*See:* Alzheimer's Disease and Dementia

# ■ DEPRESSION
*See:* Anxiety and Mood Disorders

# ■ DIABETES MELLITUS (DM)
A disease in which the body does not produce or properly use **insulin**, a **hormone** needed to convert carbohydrates (sugar, starches) and other food into energy for living. Scientists continue researching the cause of diabetes, but **genetics**, obesity, and lack of exercise appear to be factors.

## INCIDENCE
The chance of being diagnosed with diabetes has increased 61 percent among the adults in the United States since 1991; this is expected to

---

## DID YOU KNOW?

### Diabetes in People 20 Years and Older, United States

|  | 1988 to 1994 | 1999 to 2000 | 2001 to 2002 | 2003 to 2004 |
|---|---|---|---|---|
| Percentage of people 20 years and older with diabetes | 7.8 | 8.3 | 9.6 | 10.3 |

Between 1988 and 2004, the percentage of adults with diabetes rose from 7.8 percent to 10.3 percent.

Source: Centers for Disease Control and Prevention, National Center for Health Statistics, National Health and Nutrition Examination Survey, 2007.

continue in the future. There are 20.8 million people, 7 percent of the population of the United States, who have diabetes. Nearly a third of these are unaware that they have the disease. Diabetes is the sixth-leading cause of death in the United States.

The lifetime risk of diabetes for people born in the United States in 2000 is:

- for all Americans: 1 of 3 is at risk;
- for all African Americans and Hispanic males: 2 of 5; and
- for Hispanic women and girls: 1 of 2.

Diabetes affects people of all ages, sexes, and races. Statistics compiled by the Centers for Disease Control and Prevention, the National Center for Health Statistics, and the 2007 National Health and Nutrition Examination Survey indicate that African Americans suffer from diabetes more often (at 12.7 percent) than whites (at 9.2 percent) or Hispanics (at 9.3 percent). While diabetes has increased in both men and women, men still have a higher rate of diabetes. Between 1988 and 1994, almost 9 percent of men had diabetes and approximately 8 percent of women had diabetes. More recently, between 2001 and 2004, almost 12 percent of men had diabetes and approximately 9 percent of women had diabetes.

## TYPE 1 DIABETES

There are primarily two types of diabetes mellitus: Type 1 diabetes (Type 1 DM) and Type 2 diabetes (Type 2 DM). In Type 1 DM, the affected individual has a malfunction of the insulin-forming cells of the pancreas—the islets of Langerhans. It is believed to be an autoimmune disorder that starts the process, and eventually no insulin is secreted by the person's own pancreas, making the individual totally dependent upon external insulin injected into the body. This type of diabetes usually starts in childhood through young adulthood and cannot be treated with oral medications. Many people with this type of diabetes use newer insulin devices, such as insulin pens or insulin pumps, to deliver the insulin.

Between 5 and 10 percent of Americans with diabetes have Type 1 DM. Having a sibling with Type 1 diabetes and having parents with Type 1 diabetes are risk factors for getting Type 1 diabetes. Usually diagnosed in children and young adults, Type 1 diabetes may be associated with the conditions of **hyperglycemia, hypoglycemia, ketoacidosis,** or celiac disease.

Ketoacidosis is the result of protein breakdown that occurs in Type 1 DM patients when a cellular imbalance is created by inadequate insulin or the body's inability to use insulin properly. The body should maintain balanced pH values, but the ketone proteins that build up from the cellular imbalance create an acidic state that must be corrected. The patient with diabetic ketoacidosis must go to the emergency room and begin intravenous fluid and insulin and potassium replacement to correct the cellular imbalance.

Celiac disease is an autoimmune disease in which the body cannot break down foods with gluten properly. Glutens, found in wheat products, are very common in the American diet. The patient with celiac disease will have gastrointestinal symptoms, such as abdominal cramping, diarrhea, and weight loss, due to the body's inability to break down glutens.

## TYPE 2 DIABETES

In Type 2 diabetes, the most common form of the disease (90–95 percent of all diagnosed cases), the body either does not produce enough

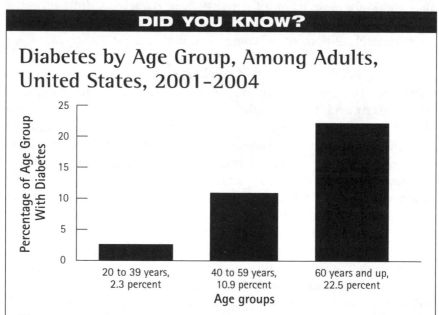

**DID YOU KNOW?**

## Diabetes by Age Group, Among Adults, United States, 2001–2004

Percentage of Age Group With Diabetes

20 to 39 years, 2.3 percent

40 to 59 years, 10.9 percent

60 years and up, 22.5 percent

Age groups

The percentage of people with diabetes increases significantly with age, from 2.3 percent before age 40 to 22.5 percent after age 60.

Source: Centers for Disease Control and Prevention, National Center for Health Statistics, National Health and Nutrition Examination Survey, 2007.

insulin or the cells resist the insulin. Normally, the body breaks down the sugars and starches that one eats into glucose, which fuels the body's cells. Insulin carries sugar from the blood into the cells. When glucose builds up in the blood instead of going into the cells it can cause two problems. The immediate one is that the cells may starve for energy. The other problem is that over time, high blood glucose levels may hurt the eyes, kidneys, nerves, or heart.

In Type 2 DM, the individual usually has insulin secretion for several years after being diagnosed with the disease. A person with Type 2 DM has metabolic factors making it harder for the body to efficiently use insulin; this requires the pancreas to produce more and more. Often, oral medications are used early in the treatment plan because they can focus on those metabolic factors. After a few years, most, but not all, patients with Type 2 DM will also require extra insulin by injection. Although having Type 2 diabetes is serious, people with it can live long, healthy lives.

## ASSOCIATED CONDITIONS

Conditions associated with Type 2 diabetes include hyperglycemia and hypoglycemia. Both Type 1 and Type 2 DM increase the risk for complications of heart disease, kidney disease, blindness, nerve damage, and amputations. The key to avoiding complications is attaining good glucose levels and controlling other risk factors aggressively.

## RISK FACTORS

Some risk factors for Type 2 DM are being over age 45, having a family history of diabetes, having one relative with the disease, and belonging to certain racial or ethnic groups (African American, Latino, Asian, Pacific Islander, and Native American). However, the biggest factors in developing Type 2 DM are controllable: obesity and being **sedentary.**

## PREVENTION AND TREATMENT

There are no known means of preventing Type 1 DM at this time, although research continues to explore this. Obesity is a major risk factor for Type 2 diabetes; more than 80 percent of people with diabetes are overweight. Recent studies have shown that people at high risk for Type 2 diabetes can prevent or delay the onset of the disease by losing 5 to 7 percent of their body weight by eating more healthfully and getting 30 minutes of physical activity five times per week.

These steps can cut the risk for developing Type 2 diabetes by nearly 60 percent.

## STEPS TO TAKE IF DIAGNOSED

First and most importantly after diagnosis, you should talk to your health-care provider to get diabetes education. This is a manageable but lifelong disease, and becoming knowledgeable will allow you to make decisions about how to eat healthfully, take medication, and prevent complications. You and your health-care provider should pay close attention to your blood glucose levels, blood pressure, and cholesterol levels during quarterly office appointments. Next, you should exercise 30 to 60 minutes most days of the week to help control blood glucose, weight, and blood pressure as well as raise your "good" cholesterol and lower your "bad" cholesterol. Exercise is also part of the next step—maintaining a healthy weight. Sometimes, early in Type 2 diabetes, eating a healthy diet with complex carbohydrates, vegetables, and lean protein while avoiding simple sugars can control blood sugars without the need for medication. If you have diabetes, you need to check your feet daily for cuts, blisters, red spots, and swelling and notify your health-care provider if you have sores that will not heal. The last step is to check your blood glucose and take the medicines your health-care provider prescribes for you.

## TREATMENT

Type 1 diabetes treatment involves injections of insulin or use of an insulin pump, careful monitoring of blood glucose levels, and regular meals and snacks to keep blood glucose levels steady. Type 2 DM can often be treated early in the diagnosis with oral medications, but the insulin supply usually needs supplementing after a few years.

## PREDIABETES

Prediabetes is a condition of blood glucose levels that are higher than normal but not yet high enough to be diagnosed as diabetes. This includes glucose levels between 110 and 126. In the United States, 54 million people have prediabetes. The long-term damage to the heart and circulatory system may already be occurring in prediabetes. On the other hand, research shows that taking action to manage your blood glucose when you have prediabetes can delay or prevent Type 2 diabetes from ever developing. This includes making diet changes and increasing one's levels of physical activity.

# TEENS SPEAK

## *Living with Diabetes*

I'm Zach and I'm 16. I was diagnosed with Type 2 diabetes last year. I had put on quite a bit of weight since I was 11. I had quit riding my bike and running around outside because I really got into video games. Eventually, I wasn't very comfortable doing those things like riding a bike, and I mostly watched television and played my games. The more I hung out around the house, the more I ate junk food.

Then last year I started drinking fluids like crazy, but I was still always thirsty. And I'd get up four or five times a night to go to the bathroom. I was so tired and got more and more hungry.

My mom has diabetes and she recognized the symptoms and took me to my doctor. She diagnosed me with Type 2 diabetes. At first my blood sugars were so high I had to inject some insulin a couple times a day. I also had to check my blood sugars by pricking my finger with a lancet several times a day. That helps the doctor and me keep my blood sugars in a safe range.

I went to a diabetes educator who taught me about this disease and how more and more kids my age are getting it. It's usually because we quit doing active stuff and start staying at home and eating more unhealthy food, so we gain weight. I got some advice on eating that was pretty simple—cut out regular sodas and juices and eat a balanced diet. I can still have an occasional treat, just not all the time.

I started exercising again—sometimes I just ride my bike around or take a walk around the block—and now I do some activity every day. I still play video games, but I balance it with some outdoor exercise. My weight has almost come back to the healthy range and I've been able to get off insulin and onto pills to treat my disease. My doctor said if I keep doing this well, I may end up on very little medicine for a while. I'm going to keep trying for that. I feel much better now than I did a year ago.

## COMPLICATIONS OF DIABETES

Heart disease and stroke, forms of **cardiovascular disease,** occur at rates two to four times higher in adults with diabetes than in those without. In 2005, 5.7 million persons aged 35 and older with diabetes reported having cardiovascular disease, a 36 percent increase from 1997.

Diabetes is a leading cause of the **chronic** kidney disease that affects 3.8 million people in the United States. Another associated disease is diabetic eye disease, in which the vessels of the eye swell and leak liquid into the **retina,** blurring the vision and sometimes leading to blindness. Diabetics are also more likely than those without diabetes to develop cataracts, a clouding of the eye's lens, and glaucoma-related optic nerve damage.

Lower-extremity amputations resulting from nerve damage, circulation problems, or infections are a serious risk for people with diabetes. Good control of blood sugars with medication and proper foot care can reduce the number of amputations.

*See also:* Chronic Disease; Genetic Disorders; Eye Disorders; Heart Disease; Obesity; Treatment

**FURTHER READING**

Bernstein, Richard. *Diabetes Solution.* New York: Little, Brown, 2007.
Drum, David, and Terry Zierenberg. *The Type 2 Diabetes Sourcebook.* 3d ed. New York: McGraw-Hill, 2006.

# ■ DOWN SYNDROME

*See:* Genetic Disorders

# ■ EATING DISORDERS

Illnesses that include extreme emotions, attitudes, and behaviors surrounding weight and food issues. Eating disorders, such as **anorexia, bulimia,** and **binge-eating disorder,** are serious emotional and physical problems that can have life-threatening consequences for both females and males.

## ANOREXIA NERVOSA

Anorexia nervosa, which is characterized by self-starvation and excessive weight loss, includes symptoms of refusal to maintain normal body weight, intense fear of weight gain, feeling overweight despite dramatic weight loss, loss of menstrual periods, and extreme concern with body weight and shape. In anorexia nervosa's self-starvation cycle, the body slows down all its processes to save energy and has these health consequences: abnormally slow heart rate and low blood pressure; increasing risk of heart failure as the heart rate and blood-pressure levels sink lower and lower; dry, brittle bones; muscle loss and weakness; severe **dehydration** that can result in kidney failure; fainting; fatigue; serious electrolyte abnormalities that could trigger heart disturbances; overall weakness; dry hair and skin; hair loss; and growth of a downy layer of hair all over body in an effort to warm the body.

# TEENS SPEAK

## *My Sister Melanie Has Anorexia*

I want to tell you about my sister, Melanie. I'm 15 and she's 16, so we've always been close—up until last year.

I was into competitive sports like basketball and softball and consider myself pretty healthy. Melanie headed more for dance and gymnastics. In those activities, the coaches and teachers can be very critical, and I know the ballet teacher told her to "lose her paunch." She came home and cried because she felt like her teacher thought she was fat. We had just been to the doctor for our appointments, and I know for sure she said Melanie was a perfect weight for her height and age. She looked normal to me, so the teacher's comment made me angry, too.

But Melanie was hurt and her self-confidence took a hit. She started dieting and lost 10 or 15 pounds. She looked a little thin to me, but not terribly unhealthy. She was getting compliments from her coaches and teachers and other kids at school, so she loved it. But she kept going.

She would eat a salad and a couple bites of meat at meals and say she was full and excuse herself while the rest of us were still eating. I became suspicious that she was vomiting, so I followed her one day. I found she was making herself vomit. I called her on it and told my parents. That was a scene, but she denied it was a problem and then promised to eat more and stop vomiting. Mom and Dad bought everything she said, but I wasn't sure.

She started changing the clothes she wore. She wore these huge clothes that hung on her and covered her up. She exercised more and more. One day I walked by her room while she was changing her clothes and her shoulders and ribs stuck out. I talked to Mom and Dad, and they agreed it was time to do something more. They took her to the doctor who confirmed she had anorexia nervosa and referred her to an outpatient treatment program at an eating-disorder clinic. She continued to lose weight and looked awful. Her hair was falling out, her color was awful, and all she cared about was exercising.

Melanie was then hospitalized for inpatient treatment. She had an IV and feedings and intensive therapy. She was angry about being hospitalized and forced to gain weight but she completed the program.

It's been two months since she's been home and she's still struggling. I wish she could see herself realistically and we could get on with our "normal" lives. But the whole family is involved in therapy and I learned it isn't that easy or fast. We will give her the support she needs to get back to a normal life one day.

## BULIMIA NERVOSA

Bulimia nervosa, a secretive cycle of binge eating followed by purging, includes eating large amounts of food—more than most people would eat in one meal—in short periods of time, then getting rid of the food and calories through vomiting, laxative abuse, or overexercising. The entire digestive system can be affected as well as electrolyte and chemical imbalances in the body that affect the heart and other major organ functions. Other health consequences include a potential for gastric rupture during bingeing periods, **inflammation** and possible rupture of the esophagus from frequent vomiting, tooth decay and staining from stomach acids released during frequent vomiting, **chronic** irregular bowel movements and constipation as a result of laxative abuse, peptic ulcers, and **pancreatitis,** inflammation or infection of the pancreas.

## BINGE-EATING DISORDER

Binge-eating disorder, also known as compulsive overeating, includes uncontrolled, impulsive, or continuous eating beyond the point of feeling comfortably full. Although there is no purging, there may be fasts, diets, and feelings of shame or self-hatred after bingeing. **Anxiety, depression,** and loneliness can contribute to the bingeing episodes. Health consequences of binge-eating disorder are the same as with clinical obesity, including high blood pressure, high **cholesterol,** heart disease due to elevated **triglyceride** levels, Type 2 diabetes, and gallbladder disease.

---

## DID YOU KNOW?

# Listen to Your Body

Eat when you are truly hungry. Stop when you are full.

- The **FIRST** key to listening to your body is being able to **detect when you are getting hungry.** If you are indeed truly hungry, and not just looking for food to cure your boredom, stress, or loneliness, then it is time to refuel.

- The **SECOND** key is being able to **know when you have had enough. Listen to your body.** When you begin to feel full, you will know that you have had enough to eat. The goal is to feel content—not uncomfortably stuffed but not starving either. For some people this means planning five or six smaller, well-balanced meals a day instead of three large meals. And remember, it takes about 20 minutes for your body to realize it's full. Also, **be aware of what you are eating**—eat sitting down, chew slowly, and enjoy the tastes, smells, and textures of your food.

- The **THIRD** key is moderation; nothing to extremes. Often people hear this advice and think it means they can eat whatever they crave, all the time. Obviously we cannot survive on potato chips or peanut butter cookies alone. And if you tried, chances are you'd probably start to crave some pasta or fresh fruit after a while. These cravings are your body's way of helping you get the nutrients it knows you need.

The keys to achieving a healthy body weight are eating when you are hungry; stopping when you are full; and eating all foods in moderation.

Source: National Eating Disorders Association, 2005.

## CAUSES OF EATING DISORDERS

People with eating disorders may use the control of food to compensate for feelings and emotions that might otherwise seem overwhelming. Dieting, bingeing, and purging may be a way to cope with powerful emotions and to feel in control of one's life, but in the end these behaviors damage a person's physical and emotional health, self-esteem, and sense of control.

Psychological factors that can contribute to an eating disorder are low self-esteem, feelings of inadequacy or lack of control, depression, anxiety, anger, or loneliness. Interpersonal factors that can contribute to eating disorders include troubled family and personal relationships, difficulty expressing emotions, a history of teasing or ridicule based on weight, and a history of physical or sexual abuse. Social factors that can contribute to an eating disorder are cultural pressure for thinness and a perfect body, narrow definitions of beauty based on preference for certain body types, and cultural values of people based on physical appearance. Scientists are still researching biological factors that contribute to eating disorders. They are finding that certain brain chemicals that control hunger, appetite, and digestion are unbalanced in those with eating disorders and that eating disorders often run in families.

## PREVENTION

Eating disorders are serious, complex problems, and physical, emotional, social, and family issues must be addressed for effective prevention and treatment. The earlier an eating disorder is discovered and addressed, the better the chance for recovery. Effective treatment programs also must address cultural obsession with thinness as a physical, psychological, and moral issue, roles of women and men in society, and development of people's self-esteem and self-respect in a variety of areas (school, work, community service, hobbies) that transcend physical appearance.

## ATHLETES AND EATING DISORDERS

In a study of Division I NCAA athletes, more than one-third of female athletes reported attitudes and symptoms placing them at risk for anorexia nervosa. Though most athletes with eating disorders are female, male athletes are also at risk—especially those competing in sports that tend to place an emphasis on the athlete's diet, appearance, size, and weight requirements.

Risk factors for athletes are sports that emphasize appearance or weight requirements such as gymnastics, diving, bodybuilding, and wrestling; sports that focus on individuals rather than the entire team;

endurance sports such as track and field sports, running, and swimming; belief that lower weight will improve performance; training for a sport since childhood or being an elite athlete; low self-esteem; family dysfunction; families with eating disorders; chronic dieting; history of physical or sexual abuse; peer, family, and cultural pressure to be thin; other traumatic life experiences; and coaches who focus only on success rather than on the athlete as a whole person.

*See also:* Anxiety and Mood Disorders; Obesity

**FURTHER READING**
Kirkpatrick, Jim, and Paul Caldwell. *Eating Disorders: Everything You Need to Know.* Buffalo, N.Y.: Firefly, 2001.
Levenkron, Steven. *Anatomy of Anorexia.* New York: W.W. Norton, 2000.

# ■ EMPHYSEMA
*See:* Chronic Obstructive Pulmonary Disease (COPD)

# ■ EPIDEMICS AND PANDEMICS
Disease outbreaks in which some or many people in a community or region become infected with the same disease. One way this can happen is by a disease being brought into the community by an outside source, such as an infected traveler returning home with the disease, or an insect carrying the disease infecting people as it bites. Another method is a **pathogen** (a **virus** or bacterium) changing in a way that enables it to evade the human **immune system,** making the pathogen stronger and more aggressive. Another way an epidemic can occur is when a new disease, such as AIDS, or a new version of an old disease, such as influenza, emerges.

For example, there are three main types of influenza viruses: A, B, and C. Influenza C causes only mild disease and has not been associated with widespread outbreaks. Influenza types A and B, however, cause epidemics nearly every year.

## PANDEMICS
An epidemic that spreads throughout the world is a pandemic, which can involve an old disease, such as smallpox or bubonic plague, or

a new form of an old disease that develops and spreads. Very few people would be resistant to a strong, new pathogen or a new form of an old pathogen. This would cause worldwide high rates of illness and death unless there is quick development and implementation of effective prevention strategies. Although its development and testing is time-intensive, a **vaccine** is an effective prevention.

## THE H1N1 PANDEMIC

In June 2009, the World Health Organization declared the H1N1 flu (often called swine flu) a pandemic, the first in 41 years. In the first two months, 74 countries reported 27,737 cases of the disease and 141 deaths. Most of the cases were in the Americas, but a dramatic rise in the number of cases in Australia and other continents led to the declaration of a pandemic. The H1N1 virus has two genes from flu viruses that occur in pigs in Europe and Asia, as well as avian and human genes. Although H1N1 appeared to be less deadly than the seasonal flu, which typically claims 30,000 lives yearly in the world, some experts speculated about the virus's possibly mutating and reappearing in a stronger form a few months later; major efforts were made to develop a vaccine before that could occur. The new H1N1 virus spreads in the same way that seasonal flu spreads—from person-to-person, through coughing and sneezing.

## PANDEMIC HISTORY

In the Spanish influenza pandemic of 1918, approximately 20 to 40 percent of the worldwide population became ill, and more than 20 million people died. In the United States alone, between September 1918 and April 1919, about 500,000 deaths occurred from the flu. The course of the disease was fast—some people who felt well in the morning were dead that same night, and the age group with the highest death rate was 20 to 50 years. No virus since that time has caused so many deaths so quickly.

The next pandemic was the Asian flu of 1957, followed by the Hong Kong flu of 1968. In 1976, there was a swine flu scare; in 1977, there was a Russian flu scare. Recent pandemic scares were the 1997 and 1999 avian flu, in which the virus moved directly from chickens to people. To prevent the virus from spreading, all chickens (1.5 million) were slaughtered in Hong Kong, where it started. Following the poultry slaughter, no new human infections were found.

Since December 2003, public health officials in Asia, Africa, and Europe have reported an increase in outbreaks of H5N1, a highly

## DID YOU KNOW?

# U.S. Preparation Strategy for Pandemic Influenza

The United States has a detailed strategic plan to prepare for pandemic influenza outbreaks.

- Intensify surveillance and collaborate on containment measures, both international and domestic

- Stockpile antiviral vaccines and work with industry to expand capacity for production of medical countermeasures

- Create a network of national, state, and local preparedness, including an increase in health-care surge capacity

- Develop the public education and communication efforts so critical to keeping the public informed—provide guidance to state and local partners as well as staffing and supplies, distribute vaccines and antiviral drugs, and assign roles and responsibilities for decision makers and community measures to control infections and limit spread of disease

- Work with the World Health Organization to improve surveillance of avian flu; provide lab assistance and training to local public health officials to detect and report H5N1 in Asia and Africa

Source. U.S. Department Health and Human Services, 2005.

pathogenic strain of avian influenza in poultry. Global agriculture has lost more than $10 billion to the disease and the livelihoods of 300 million farmers have been affected.

There has been no sustained human-to-human transmission of the H5N1 virus yet found. However, if a person were infected by the bird flu and human flu at the same time, the viruses would have the opportunity to exchanges **genes.** This process of **gene swapping** could give the virus the ability to move from human to human. Few if any people would have natural immunity, and seasonal flu vaccines would not be effective. An influenza pandemic could result in high rates of illness and death.

*See also:* Centers for Disease Control and Prevention (CDC); Immunization

**FURTHER READING**
DeSalle, Rob, ed. *Epidemic! The World of Infectious Disease.* New York: New Press, 1999.
Markel, Howard. *When Germs Travel.* New York: Pantheon, 2004.
Turkington, Carol, and Bonnie Lee Ashby. *Encyclopedia of Infectious Diseases.* New York: Facts On File, 2003.

## ■ EYE DISORDERS

Problems affecting the eyes that are often minor and temporary but may lead to permanent loss of vision. Common eye problems are cataracts, glaucoma, retinal disorders, and conjunctivitis.

Having regular eye exams is important because eye diseases do not always have symptoms. Vision loss can be prevented by early detection and treatment. Symptoms that indicate you should see an eye health-care provider immediately are changes in vision, everything appearing dim, seeing light flashes, having pain, experiencing double vision, leaking fluid from the eye, and having inflammation.

---

### DID YOU KNOW?

## People Who Have Trouble Seeing, Even with Glasses or Contacts

| Age Group | Percent of Age Group That Has Trouble Seeing |
|---|---|
| 18–24 | 5 percent |
| 25–44 | 5.6 percent |
| 45–54 | 11.7 percent |
| 55–64 | 12.7 percent |
| 65–74 | 13.6 percent |
| 75 and up | 21.7 percent |

The possibility that a person will have trouble seeing increases with age.

Source: Centers for Disease Control and Prevention, National Center for Health Statistics, National Health and Nutrition Examination Survey, 2007.

There are two basic types of eye-care professionals. Optometrists are doctors who complete eight years of study (four for a bachelor's degree, four for the doctor of optometry degree). They can examine, diagnose, treat and manage eye disorders. They can prescribe medications, lenses, and contact lenses. Ophthalmologists are medical doctors who specialize in care of the eye. They can do all that the optometrist does, but they can also perform surgery on the eye.

## CATARACTS

A cataract is a clouding of the lens in the eye that affects vision; it is related to aging. More than half of all Americans either have a cataract or have had cataract surgery by age 80. When the lens is clear, it helps focus light or an image on the **retina**, the light-sensitive tissue at the back of the eye. The lens must be clear for the retina to receive a sharp image; if the lens is cloudy, the image will be blurred. The lens is made mostly of water and protein, which is arranged in a precise way that keeps the lens clear and lets light pass through. As people age, some protein may clump together and start to cloud a small area of the lens. This is a cataract, which may grow larger and cloud more of the lens, making it harder to see. Smoking, diabetes, and prolonged exposure to sunlight are risk factors, but it may be that the protein in the lens just changes from the wear and tear it takes over the years. Some people get cataracts in their 40s and 50s, but they are small and do not affect vision; after age 60 most cataracts become noticeable.

Symptoms include cloudy or blurry vision; seeing faded colors and glare from headlights, lamps, and sunlight; seeing halos around lights; poor night vision; double vision or multiple images in one eye; and frequent prescription changes for eyeglasses or contact lenses.

Wearing sunglasses and a hat with a brim to block ultraviolet sunlight may help delay cataracts. Stopping smoking and eating nutritious foods—including green leafy vegetables, fruit, and other foods with **antioxidants**—are good preventive measures for cataracts. A comprehensive dilated eye exam at least once every two years with a check for macular degeneration, cataracts, glaucoma, and other eye disorders is recommended.

Early cataracts may be improved with new eyeglasses, brighter lighting, antiglare sunglasses, or magnifying lenses. If these do not help, surgery is the only effective treatment. Surgery involves removing the cloudy lens and replacing it with an artificial lens. A cataract needs to be removed only when vision loss interferes with everyday activities, such as driving, reading, or watching TV.

## GLAUCOMA

Glaucoma is a group of diseases that can damage the eyes' optic nerve and result in vision loss and blindness. The optic nerve, actually a bundle of more than 1 million nerve fibers, connects the retina to the brain. The optic nerve can be damaged when the normal fluid pressure inside the eyes slowly rises. As a healthy optic nerve is necessary for good vision, controlling the pressure of eye fluid is important.

Highest at risk for glaucoma are African Americans over age 40, everyone over age 60, especially Hispanics, and people with a family history of glaucoma. Among African Americans, research shows glaucoma is:

- five times more likely to occur than in Caucasians;
- four times more likely to cause blindness than in Caucasians;
- 15 times more likely to cause blindness in people aged 45–64 than Caucasians in the same age group.

### Risk Factors and Symptoms

A comprehensive dilated eye exam can reveal more risk factors, such as high eye pressure, thinness of the **cornea,** and abnormal optic nerve anatomy. In some people, medicines in the form of eyedrops can reduce the risk of developing glaucoma by about half. The best way to control the disease is early detection and treatment.

At first there are no symptoms, vision is normal, and there is no pain. As the disease progresses, a person with glaucoma may notice the gradual failing of side vision. Objects in front may still be seen clearly, but objects to the side may be missed. As the disease progresses, people may miss objects to the side and out of the corner of the eye. Without treatment, people with glaucoma will slowly lose their peripheral side vision; they seem to be looking through a tunnel. Over time, straight-ahead vision may decrease until no vision remains. Glaucoma may develop in one or both eyes.

### Detecting Glaucoma

Glaucoma is detected in five ways. A visual acuity test is an eye chart test that measures how well you see at various distances. A visual field test measures side (peripheral) vision. In a dilated eye exam, drops cause your pupil to dilate, and a magnifying lens then examines your retina and optic nerve for signs of damage and other eye problems. A test can be done for the pressure inside the eye, and another test measures the thickness of your cornea.

### Treatment
Early treatment can delay progression of the disease. Treatments include medicines, draining fluid out of the eye by laser, conventional surgery to make a new channel for the fluid to drain from the eye, or a combination of these. Although these treatments may save the remaining vision, they do not improve sight already lost from glaucoma. Medicines in the form of eyedrops or pills are the most common early treatment for glaucoma. Some medicines cause the eye to make less fluid, while others lower pressure by helping fluid drain from the eye.

## RETINAL EYE DISORDERS
There are several eye disorders that affect the retina, the layer of tissue at the back of the eye that senses light and sends images to your brain. In the center of the nerve tissue is the **macula.** It provides the sharp, central vision needed for reading, driving, and seeing fine detail. Retinal disorders affect this vital tissue. They can affect your vision and some can be serious enough to cause blindness.

## RETINAL DETACHMENT
Retinal detachment is a medical emergency when the retina is pulled away from the back of the eye. Symptoms include increase in the number of floaters, the little cobwebs or specks that float about in your field of vision, and/or light flashes in the eye. Another symptom is a curtain appearing over the field of vision. Individuals with diabetes are prone to a small vessel leaking into the retina (retinopathy), and this can cause severe vision loss if untreated.

## CONJUNCTIVITIS
Conjunctivitis is an eye infection also known as pinkeye. It can be caused by a **virus** or a bacterium and can cause red, itchy, painful eyes. Both kinds are very **contagious** and usually spread to others after the affected individuals rub their eyes, and then their hands come into contact with someone else's hand. If conjunctivitis is suspected, a healthcare provider should evaluate and treat the eyes if necessary.

**FURTHER READING**
Abel, Robert, Jr. *The Eye Care Revolution.* New York: Kensington, 1999.

---

**DID YOU KNOW?**

## Sports Eye Injuries

Almost all of the more than 40,000 sports-related eye injuries that people suffer each year can be prevented. Most sports-related eye injuries occur in baseball, basketball, and racquet sports.

To avoid eye injuries:

- In racquet sports and basketball, wear safety goggles (with protective polycarbonate lenses).
- For baseball, wear batting helmets with polycarbonate face shields.
- For hockey, use helmets and face shields approved by the U.S. Amateur Hockey Association.
- Know that standard glasses do not adequately protect the eyes.

Source: Prevent Blindness America, 2007.

---

Fekrat, Sharon, and Jennifer Weizer, eds. *All about Your Eyes.* Durham, N.C.: Duke University Press, 2006.

## ■ GENETIC DISORDERS

Disorders caused by **mutations,** or changes, in **genes** or by the rearrangement of genes on **chromosomes.** Genes carry DNA, which contains the hereditary information determining an individual's characteristics. Children inherit the changed or rearranged information of genetic disorders from their parents. **Congenital** genetic disorders are present at birth, while other genetic disorders appear later in life. There are three basic kinds of genetic disorders:

(1) disorders caused by a mutation, or change, to a single gene (for example, cystic fibrosis and color blindness);

(2) disorders caused by abnormalities in whole chromosomes, which contain many genes (as in **Down syndrome**); and

(3) disorders caused by an interaction of genes and the environment (as in diabetes and high blood pressure).

## CYSTIC FIBROSIS

Cystic fibrosis (CF) is an inherited **chronic** disease affecting the lungs and digestive system. The approximately 30,000 people in the United States with cystic fibrosis have a defective gene. This gene makes a protein that causes the body to produce unusually thick, sticky mucus. The mucus clogs the lungs and intestines and leads to life-threatening lung infections.

Unusually high in salt, the mucus of people with cystic fibrosis is thicker and stickier than normal mucus, making it harder for the **respiratory** system to push it up and out. The airways become blocked. People with this disease cough a great deal because their bodies are trying to clear the passageways. If the passageways are not clear, **alveoli**, the final branches of the lung tree where carbon dioxide and oxygen are enlarged, can get inflamed, making it even harder to breathe. If the condition worsens, the lungs can collapse.

Another problem with salty mucus is that it makes it harder for the body's white blood cells to find and kill the germs that make their way down into the respiratory system, leading to chronic infections. People with cystic fibrosis have an additional problem with respiratory infections because the body's natural response is to produce more mucus, which actually makes the problem worse.

In the digestive system, the thick mucus creates a different problem. It clogs the small tubes leading out of the pancreas. Normally, the pancreas produces about 32 ounces of **enzymes** a day. With the pancreatic tubes blocked, the enzymes that would normally break down food in the stomach never get to their destination. Eventually, the pancreas can become scarred and may stop producing enzymes as well as it used to; sometimes it leads to pancreatitis. Instead of nourishing the body, the food passes out of the body as unused waste. People with cystic fibrosis also cannot reabsorb the salt they sweat out, so they become dehydrated faster than other people.

### Cystic Fibrosis Is Inherited

In 1989, scientists discovered that cystic fibrosis is caused by a problem with a gene on chromosome 7 of the 23 pairs of chromosomes that humans have. More than 10 million Americans are **carriers** of the defective gene; they do not have symptoms of the disease, but they have one defective gene and can pass along that gene to a child. If the other parent also has the defective gene, and the child inherits one defective gene from each parent, the child will have the disease.

### Genetic Testing

Genetic testing can identify three out of four people with cystic fibrosis. A DNA test for the defective gene is performed on cells scraped from the inside of the cheeks. To confirm the diagnosis, a sweat test is often done as well. People with cystic fibrosis have two to five times the sweat of people without the disease.

## Fact Or Fiction?

### If two carriers have a child, the child will have cystic fibrosis.

**The Facts:** If two carriers have a child, there is a one-in-four, or 25 percent, chance that the child will have cystic fibrosis. There is a 50 percent chance the child will be a carrier and a 25 percent chance that the child will not inherit a defective gene and, thus, will not be a carrier. About one out of every 30 white Americans is a carrier of cystic fibrosis. One out of every 3,600 babies is born with cystic fibrosis.

### Treatment

Treatments and therapies can vary by case. Because cystic fibrosis affects the lungs, much of the treatment focuses on clearing mucus from the airways. Once the mucus is loosened from the airways, it can be coughed out. Aerobic exercise is helpful for expanding the lungs' capacity to hold more air, making the body more efficient at getting oxygen out of the air, and for keeping infections out of the lungs. Medications used to treat cystic fibrosis include: mucus thinners that make the mucus easier to cough out; **antibiotics** to kill or slow **bacteria**; **anti-inflammatories** to reduce **inflammation** and swelling of body tissues; bronchodilators to open the airways for easier breathing; and pancreatic enzymes to help digest food.

### Gene Therapy

As scientists continue to learn more about cystic fibrosis and experiment with new drugs and therapies, the outlook for the future is positive. Since the isolation of the gene responsible for cystic fibrosis in 1989, the possibility of **gene therapy** has opened up. Gene therapy is the replacement of defective genes with normal genes. Although scientists have been able to change the genes of cells in the laboratory, they are still working on solving the problem of changing genes in lung cells of people with cystic fibrosis. Because **viruses** can get inside cells, scientists are experimenting with using viruses to deliver the gene therapy.

This method has its problems, however. Often the patient's body attacks the virus delivering the gene therapy because it registers the virus as dangerous. It also attacks the cells that the virus infects, the very cells that need to be saved. In addition, cells in the human body regularly die and are replaced, so the "corrected" cells die and are replaced by ones with the original genetic defect. This means that gene therapy would have to be repeated every few months so there would be enough cells with the correct information to keep the person healthy.

### Coping

Ultimately, this disease is fatal—however, people with cystic fibrosis are living longer and healthier lives than they used to. People with it need to take special care of themselves, but they can do all the things that other people do.

One way that the disease impacts the lives of sufferers is that they need to take a lot of medications and may need to carry extra pills with them, just in case they need them. They also need to have **physiotherapy** every day, so if they travel, alternative plans need to be made. Physiotherapy, usually done twice a day, helps keep the lungs clear of mucus. With the patient lying in a position that allows gravity to drain the lungs, the therapist thumps areas of the chest to loosen mucus. There are tools for performing self-physiotherapy.

Cystic fibrosis is also a concern for people who plan to have kids. Having a child means taking the risk of having a child with cystic fibrosis. Although men with the disease tend to be infertile, adoption is a problem if parents with CF worry about being healthy enough to provide all the child care needed.

## MUSCULAR DYSTROPHY

**Muscular dystrophy**, or MD, is an inherited disease that causes severe muscle weakness and progressive crippling but no neural or sensory effects. There are at least nine types of muscular dystrophy, and the types are caused by different genetic mechanisms. Exactly how these genetic disorders cause the progressive muscle weakening is not known.

Some of the forms of MD start in childhood, some during young adulthood, and others in old age. Some break down muscles quickly, while others take a long time. Different forms of MD also affect different parts of the body.

Some types of MD affect vital organs and lead to severe disability and even death. Early in the disease, muscle fiber tissues die and regenerate. Over time, regeneration slows and degeneration dominates. Weakness results when muscle fibers are replaced with fat and connective tissue. Complications can include deforming of the skeletal system, muscle weakness around the lungs inhibiting lung function and increasing the risk of pneumonia, respiratory infections, and heart problems (sudden heart failure may cause death).

## SICKLE-CELL DISEASE

Sickle-cell disease (or sickle cell disease) is an inherited congenital disease resulting from a defective **hemoglobin** molecule that causes the red blood cells to be sickle-shaped. The cells impair circulation because they are rigid rather than round and flexible like normal cells. When the sickle cells block blood vessels, it can be very painful and cause permanent damage to the bones, nervous system, and some organs. Chronic ill health results. Periodic crises, long-term complications, and premature death can occur.

### Symptoms

Symptoms include all those of anemia, such as fatigue, breathlessness, and dizziness, as well as joint pain. One common problem with sickle-cell anemia is bone pain. Like all living tissue, bones need a blood supply. They have tiny spaces in spongy areas for blood to move instead of arteries and veins. With sickle-cell anemia, the cells get trapped in the rigid, tiny areas causing the bones and **joints** to ache. The bone pain can last for several days and be quite intense. Patients usually require strong pain medication.

### Inheritance

Most common in people of African descent and in Africans who live in the tropics, worldwide about one in 10 blacks carries the abnormal gene. If two such carriers have children, each child has a one-in-four chance of developing the disease. Overall, one in every 400 to 600 black children has sickle-cell anemia. The disease also occurs in Puerto Rico, Turkey, India, the Middle East, and the Mediterranean region.

Two pairs of normal genes direct the manufacturing of the two parts of the normal hemoglobin molecule. People with sickle-cell anemia have inherited a mutated hemoglobin gene from each parent that carries faulty instructions for making half of the hemoglobin molecule. As a result, their bodies make sickle-shaped hemoglobin. The difference in sickle-shaped and normal hemoglobin is in just one of the 574 amino acids of which they are made. The mutation of the gene causes the amino acid's chemical code to be slightly changed, which directs the manufacture of the sickle-shaped hemoglobin.

Sickle-shaped hemoglobin is red and can carry oxygen just like normal hemoglobin. Problems occur when the sickle-shaped hemoglobin releases oxygen. The sickle hemoglobin forms a crystal rather than liquid inside the cell. The crystals join together into small cords and then chains that twist together. This makes the sickle cells inflexible, as opposed to the liquid, flexible shapes of normal red blood cells. The sickle cells do not easily move through the blood vessels. They stick to each other and to the sides of vessels; they pile up to form roadblocks within vessels, so the body parts beyond the blocked vessels do not receive their oxygen, food, infection fighters, protein, and fluid. Lack of oxygen causes the affected part of the body to produce chemicals that cause pain. Oxygen reverses the sickling process, causing the sickle-shaped hemoglobin to change from crystal to liquid. The sickling damages the cell membrane of the red blood cells, and after a few sicklings, or a prolonged one, the cell may be permanently sickled.

## Treatment

Medications can ease pain and fight infections associated with sickle-cell anemia, while blood transfusions and oxygen can help in emergencies. Oxygen will reverse the sickling process and cause the hemoglobin sickle to change from a crystal back to a liquid, but if the blockage remains for a very long time, tissues, deprived of supplies, will be damaged. The blockage and pain can happen anywhere in the body, sometimes in several areas at once.

A person with sickle-cell disease may suffer frequent aches and pains of sickling blockage, which can be taken care of with heating pads, fluids, rest, and ordinary painkillers. But severe pain, fever, and swelling signal a sickling crisis, and the person must go to the hospital for strong painkillers and other treatment. It is believed that infection, **dehydration,** cold weather, overexertion, or stressors such as anger or fear set the stage for a sickling crisis. For most people, sickling crises are few, but about 15 percent of people with sickle-cell disease will have three or more major pain crises a year. Each time, tissue and organs can be damaged. The greater the number of crises per year, the greater chance of dying young.

## DOWN SYNDROME

Down syndrome is a genetic disorder in which people have abnormal mental and physical development causing developmental disabilities and distinctive physical features. Some of these distinctive features include short fingers, slanted eyes, and deeply creased palms.

The leading cause of mental retardation, Down syndrome occurs in every race and economic level. In the United States each year, 4,000 babies are born with the syndrome (a set of features that together point to a condition), and more than 350,000 people with Down syndrome live in the United States.

### Testing for Down Syndrome

Doctors usually test for Down syndrome in older pregnant women, women with older husbands, or mothers who already have a Down syndrome child. A blood test indicates the risk of a child having Down syndrome by telling whether the fetus has any of three possible signs outside the normal range. If any of the three signs is outside the normal range, additional tests can be done to determine whether the syndrome is present.

### Symptoms

Some babies are born healthy and show few outward features of the condition, while others display many signs. The number of physical features displayed does not reflect someone's level of intelligence. Every person with Down syndrome is unique, as is every person without the condition.

While they are unique, people with Down syndrome share a certain physical appearance. Their heads can be smaller than normal, and they can have folds in the back of a short neck at birth. There can also be larger than normal soft spots in the skull where bones take longer to close. Both the folds and soft spots may disappear with age.

Other physical signs include eye openings that slant upward on the outside; outer ears that may be smaller, misshapen, or set lower on the head; smaller, flatter noses; smaller mouths; unique tooth problems; short, thick hands and feet; fifth fingers on each hand that curve inward; weak muscles at birth; and weak joints, especially at the top two backbones of the neck. With these weak joints there is a greater chance that stress on the head or neck will damage the spine. Although it can be corrected with surgery when the child is older, doctors advise children with this surgery to avoid heavy physical activities to prevent further stress on joints, muscle tissue, and the spine.

Although they learn more slowly than normal children, children with Down syndrome learn to sit, walk, talk, and take care of themselves. About four in five people with Down syndrome have some mental retardation. Because they are slower to observe things around them, and because they sleep more due to health problems, Down syndrome infants miss out on contact and stimulation, causing them to learn more slowly and to need more practice to learn new skills.

Problems that can accompany the disorder are vision problems, including the development of cataracts; hearing loss that prevents building language skills; heart disease resulting in fatigue; and digestion problems. Caused by a misfiring of normal electric charges in the brain, seizures as small as a blink or as serious as a total loss of body control that last from a few seconds to a few minutes are common in children with Down syndrome.

Because they age earlier than the general population, people with Down syndrome can have wrinkled skin and gray or white hair when they are in their 20s. People with Down syndrome can get **dementia,** which eventually results in memory loss, and Alzheimer's disease, a fatal brain disease causing memory loss and an inability to perform daily activities, 20 to 30 years earlier than people in the general population.

## Inheritance

Normally, in a healthy human there are 46 chromosomes in every cell, which carry genes that provide the DNA necessary for building living organisms. The chromosomes are arranged into 23 pairs, which scientists have numbered from 1 to 23. One chromosome of each pair is from the mother, and one is from the father. During cell division, the chromosomes copy themselves so that the new cell will have the exact same copies of the chromosomes of the "old" cells. In people with Down syndrome, the chromosome copy ends up with an extra 47th chromosome in each cell.

Scientists now think that more than one gene might cause Down syndrome. The heart defects, bone problems, cataracts, and other signs of early aging that often accompany Down syndrome may be caused by different genes.

# Q & A

**Question: What are the risks for older parents of having a baby with Down syndrome?**

**Answer:** Scientists continue to study why older parents are at greater risk of having a baby with Down syndrome. For 20-year-old mothers, the risk of having a baby with Down syndrome is one in 2,000. For mothers over 40, the risk is one in 100 and is even higher for mothers over 45. Although the link between a father's age and the risk of having a Down syndrome child requires more study, some scientists theorize that fathers over 50 have a greater risk than those under 50.

## Coping

Structured programs to help improve Down syndrome babies' physical, mental, and social abilities are begun as soon after birth as possible. Health-care providers can show parents exercises that are individualized to suit their child's strengths and weaknesses. When Down syndrome children reach school age, they can attend a wide range of classes with nondisabled or disabled students for all or part of the day, with or without an assistant teacher or another special education teacher. Federal law guarantees that all children receive preparation that enables them to play useful roles in the community. The Americans with Disabilities Act of 1990, an extension of the Rehabilitation Act of 1973, ensures that people beyond school age with disabilities have equal rights to public housing, transportation, and state and local government services.

## Adults with Down Syndrome

As adults, people with Down syndrome have a variety of interests, skills, and talents. Some may go to college; most find jobs—a full- or part-time regular job, supported employment with ongoing help on the job, or sheltered employment, where work is performed with others who also have disabilities.

*See also:* Anemia; Alzheimer's Disease and Dementia; Chronic Disease

**FURTHER READING**

Bellenir, Karen, ed. *Genetic Disorders Sourcebook: Basic Consumer Health Information about Hereditary Diseases and Disorders*. Detroit: Omnigraphics, 2004.

Harris, Jacqueline. *Sickle-Cell Disease*. Brookfield, Conn.: Twenty-first Century Books, 2001.

## ■ GLAUCOMA

*See*: Eye Disorders

## ■ HEART DISEASE

The leading cause of death in the United States. The beginning of coronary heart disease is a slow buildup of fat, cholesterol, and

## DID YOU KNOW?

# The Five Leading Causes of Death, United States

Deaths per 100,000 People Each Year

|  | 1990 | 1960 | 1970 | 1980 | 1990 | 2000 | 2004 |
|---|---|---|---|---|---|---|---|
| Heart disease | 568.8 | 559.0 | 492.7 | 412.1 | 321.8 | 257.6 | 217.0 |
| Cancer | 193.9 | 193.9 | 198.6 | 207.9 | 216.0 | 199.6 | 185.8 |
| Stroke | 180.7 | 177.9 | 144.7 | 96.2 | 65.2 | 60.9 | 50.0 |
| Chronic lower respiratory diseases |  |  |  | 28.3 | 37.2 | 44.2 | 41.1 |
| Unintentional injuries | 78.0 | 62.3 | 60.1 | 46.4 | 36.5 | 34.9 | 37.7 |

Although the rate of heart disease has decreased, it is still the leading cause of death.

Source: Centers for Disease Control and Prevention, National Center for Health Statistics, *Health, United States*, 2007 edition.

other substances to create **plaque,** a soft substance against the blood vessel walls of the heart. This is called **arteriosclerosis.** The spectrum of heart or **cardiovascular disease** can go from some minor plaque buildup, which gives symptoms of angina, commonly known as chest pain, to complete blockage of the heart vessels, which causes cell death in the heart, or a heart attack. Early recognition of signs and symptoms of heart disease is the key to preventing a heart attack.

## HEART ATTACK

Coronary arteries carry blood with oxygen to supply the heart muscle. A heart attack occurs when the blood flow to the heart is severely reduced or stopped. A slow buildup of fat, cholesterol, and other substances called plaque can clog the arteries. This process is called arteriosclerosis.

If a plaque breaks and a blood clot forms around it, the clot can block the flow of blood to the heart, starving the heart for oxygen and nutrients. This can result in the damage or death of part of the heart, called a myocardial infarction (MI).

### Symptoms

Although some heart attacks are sudden and intense, leaving no doubt about what is happening, most start slowly, with mild pain or discomfort. Signs of heart attack are:

- discomfort in the center of the chest that lasts more than a few minutes; a feeling of uncomfortable pressure, squeezing, fullness, or pain
- discomfort in one or both arms, the back, neck, jaw, or stomach
- shortness of breath
- breaking out in a cold sweat, nausea, or lightheadedness

Chest pain or discomfort is the most common heart attack symptom for both men and women. However, women experience some of the other symptoms, mostly shortness of breath, nausea/vomiting, and back or jaw pain more often than men, which is why it can be more difficult for them to realize that a heart attack is occurring.

## Healing

The time between the injury to the heart muscle and treatment, and the size of the heart area supplied by the damaged, blocked artery, both determine the amount of permanent damage to the heart. As the heart muscle heals in about eight weeks, scar tissue forms, and the undamaged part of the heart keeps working, although it is weaker and does not pump as much blood as before the attack.

## Treatment

Treatment for heart attacks includes medications, lifestyle changes, and interventions to the inside of the artery vessels through a wire threaded from the groin.

Medications are available for preventing clots from enlarging; preventing clots from forming; treating high blood pressure; preventing future attacks by decreasing heart rate and cardiac output, which lowers blood pressure and makes the heart beat more slowly with less force; regulating heartbeats; increasing the force of heart contractions; easing chest pain by dilating vessels; and lowering bad cholesterol, raising good cholesterol, and reducing vessel **inflammation**.

Surgical options for the treatment of heart attacks also exist. Tubes can be threaded up to the coronary arteries to widen blocked areas where blood flow to the heart has been cut off or blocked. A stent can be implanted to prop the artery open and decrease the chances of another blockage. Blocked arteries can be treated by creating a new passage for blood flow to the heart. Grafting, or taking arteries or veins from other parts of body, can reroute the blood around clogged artery. A nonfunctioning heart valve can be replaced with a healthy one. A healthy heart can be transplanted to replace a diseased heart. Skeletal muscles taken from the back or abdomen can be wrapped around an ailing heart. The heart's pumping motion can be boosted by stimulation from a device similar to a pacemaker.

Lifestyle changes include reducing cholesterol, reducing excess weight, and increasing physical activity to 30 minutes five days a week. Patients should eat a healthy diet with plenty of fruits and vegetables, high fiber, and low-fat protein with minimal trans fat and sweets. Stopping smoking and avoiding secondhand smoke are important, as is controlling diabetes if one has it.

## Risk Factors for Heart Disease

Some risk factors are unavoidable. Increasing age, being male, and having a family history of heart disease are risk factors that cannot be changed. Other risk factors can be controlled. Tobacco smoking makes the risk of developing heart disease two to four times higher than it is for nonsmokers.

High blood cholesterol (especially LDL or "bad" cholesterol) also increases the risk. Cholesterol is a soft, waxy substance that cells need to perform their functions. It comes from food eaten but also is made by the liver. You need some cholesterol for the cells, but it becomes a risk factor for plaque buildup and heart disease if the levels are too high. High blood pressure causes the heart to thicken and become less flexible, so it will not function properly.

Physical inactivity can be problematic. A **sedentary** lifestyle, one of sitting more than walking or moving about, is a risk factor. Regular moderate to vigorous physical exercise is recommended for heart health.

Obesity also presents risks. Excess body fat, especially if much of it is at the waist, is a risk factor for developing heart disease. Overweight people can lower their risk by losing as few as 10 pounds.

Diabetes mellitus is a risk factor as well. Working with a health-care provider to control blood-sugar levels will reduce the risk of heart disease in people with diabetes. At least 65 percent of people with diabetes die of a form of heart or blood vessel disease.

Stress can lead to elevated risk. Studies show that some people's reaction to stress, such as overeating, smoking, or high blood pressure, can put them at risk for heart disease.

Drinking too much alcohol can raise blood pressure, cause heart failure, and lead to strokes. It also contributes to obesity, which is in itself a risk factor.

A nutritious diet is a key factor in avoiding heart disease. The amount and type of food eaten affects other controllable risk factors such as obesity, diabetes, blood pressure, and cholesterol. A suggested diet includes vegetables, fruits, whole grains, high-fiber foods, lean proteins, and fat-free and low-fat dairy products.

## HYPERTENSION

High blood pressure was listed as the primary or a contributing cause of death in 300,000 of 2.4 million deaths in the United States in 2004.

When the heart beats, it pumps blood to the arteries and creates pressure in them. Blood pressure results from two forces: First, force is created as blood pumps into the arteries and through the circulatory system; second, a force is created as the arteries resist the blood flow. Healthy arteries are muscular and elastic, and they stretch when blood flows through them. The amount of stretching is based on how much force the blood exerts.

Blood pressure is reported as two numbers with a line between them. The higher number represents the pressure when the heart is beating, while the lower number represents the pressure when the heart is resting between beats. Normally, for an adult, blood pressure should be less than 120/80 mm Hg (millimeters of mercury). Adults with blood pressure of 140/90 mm Hg or above have hypertension and are at higher risk for heart disease, stroke, and other medical problems.

### Detecting Hypertension (High Blood Pressure)

Because there are no symptoms of high blood pressure, adults need to get their blood pressure checked each time they see their health-care provider. Although one in three—or 73 million—adults over 20 in the United States has high blood pressure, estimates are that 30 percent of them are unaware of the problem.

It is very important to become aware of blood pressure readings because high blood pressure can add to the heart and arteries' workload and enlarge the heart. The higher the blood pressure is, the greater the risk of heart attack, heart failure, stroke, and kidney disease.

### Risk Factors

Uncontrollable risk factors for hypertension include age, heredity, and race. High blood pressure occurs most often in people over 35, and the older a person gets, the greater the chance of developing high blood pressure. A person is more likely to develop it if his or her parents or other close blood relatives have high blood pressure. African Americans develop high blood pressure more often than whites and it tends to occur earlier and be more severe. More than 40 percent of African Americans have high blood pressure.

Controllable risk factors include obesity, eating too much salt, consuming too much alcohol, inactivity, and stress. People with a **body mass index (BMI)** of 30.0 or higher are more likely to develop

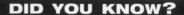

**DID YOU KNOW?**

## Hypertension and Elevated Blood Pressure Among Persons 20 Years and Older, United States, 2004

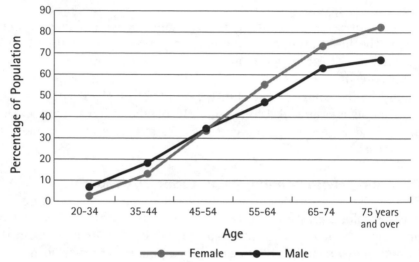

The percentage of people with hypertension increases with age, from less than 10 percent under age 34 to more than 60 percent for men and more than 80 percent for women over age 75.

Source: Centers for Disease Control and Prevention, 2007.

hypertension. Some people have increased blood pressure with high salt intake. Regular heavy use of alcohol can radically raise blood pressure. Lack of exercise can lead to obesity, which increases the risk of high blood pressure. Stress could be a factor in some people; it is hard to measure, and responses to it vary widely.

Lifestyle changes that can help regulate high blood pressure include maintaining a normal weight, using less salt, becoming more physically active, limiting alcohol consumption, and taking medications as prescribed by a health-care provider. Medications usually prescribed for controlling high blood pressure are diuretics to rid the body of excess salt and water; beta blockers to reduce heart rate and the heart's output of blood, which lowers blood pres-

---

**DID YOU KNOW?**

## Prevalence of High Blood Pressure

Among people with high blood pressure:

| Percentage with blood pressure under control | Percentage with blood pressure not under control |
|:---:|:---:|
| 35.1 percent | 64.9 percent |

Of all people with high blood pressure, about two-thirds do not have their blood pressure under control.

Source: American Heart Association, 2008.

---

sure; and drugs to open up the narrowed blood vessels and lower blood pressure. Although the cause of most cases of high blood pressure is unknown, high blood pressure is easy to detect and usually controllable.

**FURTHER READING**

Lipsky, Martin S., and Marla Mendelson. *American Medical Association Guide to Preventing and Treating Heart Disease: Essential Information*. Hoboken, N.J.: Wiley, 2008.

Otelio, Randall, and Deborah S. Romaine. *The Encyclopedia of the Heart and Heart Disease*. New York: Facts On File, 2005.

## ■ HEPATITIS

Inflammation or irritation of the liver. The liver performs more than 100 functions, many of them essential for life. One of the most important functions the liver performs is filtering some of the body's waste and removing external products such as food, medications, and alcohol. The hepatitis viruses A, B, C, D, E, and G usually cause hepatitis, but the disease can also have nonviral causes, primarily, excessive use of alcohol or drugs.

Hepatitis that lasts fewer than six months is considered **acute**; hepatitis that lasts longer than six months is considered **chronic**.

There are several types of hepatitis, but the three of the most common are A, B, C.

## TYPE A HEPATITIS

About 40 percent of hepatitis cases in the United States result from the hepatitis A virus. The number of cases is rising in people with HIV because they have susceptible **immune systems.** Type A hepatitis is highly **contagious;** the virus is often spread through human feces, usually the result of poor hygiene. Hepatitis A usually results from ingestion of contaminated food, milk, or water. Outbreaks of this type are often traced to eating seafood from polluted water. When you hear of hepatitis outbreaks related to food sources at restaurants or with produce, it is usually from Type A hepatitis. Symptoms include feeling tired or run-down, nausea, vomiting, fever above 100.4°F, and pain under the right lower rib cage. Later, the urine changes to a dark color and **jaundice** can occur. Jaundice is a yellow color change in the skin or whites of the eyes.

The severity of the hepatitis infection depends on the person's age. Children often have no symptoms and adults usually feel mildly ill, although it can be severe enough to require hospitalization or cause liver failure or death. There is no cure but to rest and to let the disease run its course. One should avoid alcohol and some prescriptions that are processed through the liver.

## TYPE B HEPATITIS

Hepatitis B is spread by blood and body fluid contact. Also increasing among HIV-positive people, hepatitis B is considered a sexually trans-mitted disease because of its high incidence and rate of transmission by this route. Screening of donated blood for the hepatitis B **antigen** has decreased cases of people getting hepatitis through transfusions. Sharing of needles by drug users, though, remains a major way of spreading the virus.

Formerly, hepatitis B was thought to be transmitted only through the exchange of contaminated blood. Now, because health-care workers are frequently exposed to hepatitis B, most hospitals offer the hepatitis B **vaccine** to their staffs at no charge to minimize the risk of infection.

The symptoms of hepatitis B are similar to those of hepatitis A. However, it is a more serious problem. About 1 million people die each year from hepatitis B. In addition to the preventive vaccine, there is a vaccine for those who know they were exposed to someone with the disease but have not yet developed the illness.

However, prevention is key. Doctors recommend that pregnant women who might transmit it during pregnancy or birth be tested. People should observe skin and body-fluid protection with use of condoms during intercourse and avoiding the sharing of articles such as toothbrushes and razors. Of course, one should not share IV needles with others and should carefully check out a tattoo shop before considering getting a tattoo, as this is also a method of transmission.

## TYPE C HEPATITIS

Primarily transmitted through blood and body fluids or obtained through tattooing, Type C accounts for 20 percent of all viral hepatitis cases. Type C is a blood-borne illness transmitted primarily by sharing of needles by drug users, unsanitary tattooing, and blood transfusions. Type C hepatitis causes 80 percent of post-transfusion hepatitis now. Fifty to 80 percent of infected people develop chronic infection. People with chronic hepatitis C are **infectious**. Hepatitis C is the most frequent cause of chronic liver disease and the most frequent disease requiring liver transplantation in the United States. The symptoms are similar to the other types of hepatitis, but the majority of cases have no symptoms.

## TYPE D HEPATITIS

Hepatitis D occurs only in people already infected with hepatitis B. In the United States, Type D is confined to people who are frequently exposed to blood and blood products, such as IV drug users and hemophiliacs.

## TYPE E HEPATITIS

Type E occurs primarily in people who have recently returned from India, Africa, Asia, or Central America. It is transmitted through absorption in the intestines, and it is usually waterborne. It is more common in young adults and more severe in pregnant females.

## TYPE G HEPATITIS

Discovered in 1995, the Type G virus is blood-borne. It usually occurs in those who receive blood transfusions.

## DID YOU KNOW?

# Preventing the Spread of Viral Hepatitis

- Thoroughly and frequently wash hands for 15–30 seconds.
- Do not share food, eating utensils, or toothbrushes.
- If you have hepatitis B, C, D, or G, do not have sexual relations or donate blood while infected. Transmission occurs through exchange of blood or body fluids that contain blood.
- Wash hands after changing a diaper or touching any soiled item.
- Wash hands before and after preparing food and eating, after going to the bathroom, and after handling garbage or dirty laundry.
- Do not drink raw (unpasteurized) milk.
- Wash raw vegetables thoroughly before eating.
- Used bagged salad as soon as possible.
- Keep raw meat separate from other foods.
- Wash hands, knives, and cutting boards after handling uncooked food.
- Thoroughly cook raw food from animal sources.
- Consider the hepatitis A vaccine for children 12–23 months of age, travelers to countries where hepatitis A is common, illegal drug users, men who have sex with men, people with chronic liver disease, adults with blood-clotting factor disorders, and adults at risk for infection at work, including day-care staff, nursing-home workers, and food handlers.

Source: National Women's Health Information Center, 1992.

## RECOVERING FROM HEPATITIS

Complete recovery takes time. The liver takes three weeks to regenerate cells and up to four months to return to normal functioning. The liver often enlarges with hepatitis. Patients are told to avoid contact sports until the liver returns to normal size to avoid bleeding or rupture of the liver. The liver is highly vascular and is usually protected by the rib cage. When it is enlarged, it is outside the protection of the rib cage and is even more vulnerable to bleeding because of the enlargement.

Good nutrition is key in helping the liver to regenerate. The Mayo Clinic recommends a high-calorie, nutrient-dense diet with fresh fruits and vegetables and whole grains. Drink adequate fluids every day. Abstain from alcohol while you have the disease to avoid additional stress on the liver. Patients should also check with their health-care provider before taking any medication, even prescribed medication and over-the-counter drugs, because many common drugs, such as acetaminophen, are processed through the liver.

*See also:* AIDS (Acquired Immunodeficiency Syndrome); Alcoholism; Immunization; Infections, Bacterial and Viral; Sexually Transmitted Diseases (STDs)

**FURTHER READING**
Hayhurst, Chris. *Everything You Need to Know about Hepatitis.* New York: Rosen, 2003.
Worman, Howard J. *The Liver Disorders and Hepatitis Sourcebook.* New York: McGraw-Hill, 2006.

# ■ HYPERTENSION
*See*: Heart Disease

# ■ IMMUNIZATION
The use of **vaccines** to strengthen the **immune system's** response to disease. Centers for Disease Control and Prevention (CDC) guidelines stress that disease prevention is key to good public health, and prevention is much easier than treatment of disease once it is contracted. Vaccines help prevent infectious diseases and save lives. Vaccines have helped to control diseases such as polio, measles, whooping cough, mumps, and tetanus, which were once prevalent in the United States.

## Immunization for Infants
Vaccines are **antigens** that have been deactivated to make them safe. The vaccines provoke an immune system response to make it ready to fight the same antigens again in the future. Immunizations, also

# Immunization Schedule for Children from Birth Through Six Years

| Vaccine | Diseases/Notes | At Age |
| --- | --- | --- |
| DTaP | diphtheria (bacterial disease), tetanus (lockjaw, a bacterial disease), pertussis (whooping cough) | 2, 4, 6, 15–18 mos., 4–6 yrs. (5 doses) |
| Hepatitis A | acute liver disease | 12–23 mos., 6 mos. later |
| Hepatitis B | a serious liver disease; chronic infection more common in children than adults | birth, 1–2, 6–18 mos. (3 doses) |
| Hib | *Haemophilus influenzae* type b: can lead to meningitis, pneumonia, blood infections | 2, 4, 6, 12–15 mos. (4 doses) |
| MMR | measles, mumps, and rubella | 12–15 mos., 4–6 yrs. |
| Pneumococcal | can lead to meningitis, blood infections, ear infections, pneumonia, deafness | 2, 4, 6, 12–15 mos. (4 doses) |
| Polio | can lead to paralysis contracted by close contact with infected person | 2, 4, 6–18 mos., 4–6 yrs. (4 doses) |
| Rotavirus | most common cause of diarrhea in children | 2, 4, 6 mos. (3 doses) |
| Varicella | chickenpox | 12–15 mos., 4–6 yrs. |

Source: Centers for Disease Control and Prevention, 2009.

called **vaccinations,** are given through pills or shots and provide people with immunity to certain diseases. Laws require certain vaccinations to protect children against diseases, and people must have vaccinations before traveling to certain countries due to diseases that are common to those areas.

Six vaccines are recommended for babies between birth and six months of age.

## IMMUNIZATIONS FOR PRETEENS AND ADOLESCENTS

The CDC and American Academy of Pediatrics recommend that preteens get these vaccines when they are 11 or 12 years old.

- Tdap vaccine: Tetanus, diphtheria, acellular pertussis (pertussis is whooping cough, which is highly **contagious**), as a booster shot.

- MCV4 vaccine: Meningococcal meningitis is an infection of the lining around the brain and spinal cord; it can cause death. Meningococcal bloodstream infection can cause loss of arms and legs and even death.

- HPV vaccine for girls: Human papillomavirus is a common **virus** in female teens and women in their 20s; it is a major cause of cervical cancer in women. It is recommended that girls get three doses of the vaccine before their first sexual contact, when they could be exposed to HPV.

## VACCINES NEEDED BY TEENS AND COLLEGE STUDENTS

Vaccines for preteens and adolescents prevent serious, sometimes life-threatening diseases. As children get older, immunity provided by some childhood vaccines can decrease, so another dose of the vaccine may be needed. Also, teens are at greater risk for diseases such as meningitis and HPV.

- tetanus-diptheria-pertussis vaccine
- meningococcal vaccine (recommended for previously unvaccinated college freshmen living in dorms)
- HPV vaccine series
- hepatitis B vaccine series
- polio vaccine series

- measles-mumps-rubella (MMR) vaccine series
- varicella (chicken pox) vaccine series
- influenza vaccine
- pneumococcal polysaccharide (PPV) vaccine
- hepatitis A vaccine series

### VACCINE-PREVENTABLE ADULT DISEASES

For adults, doctors recommend a number of vaccines for especially serious, but preventable, diseases. These include:

- **Diphtheria:** Vaccination is recommended if you have not had a booster shot in 10 years or more, or if you never had the initial three-shot series.

- **Influenza (flu):** Vaccination is recommended if you are over age 50; you are living in a nursing home; have a **chronic** disease; have immune system diseases; you are a health-care provider; you will be pregnant during flu season; you live with children under five years of age; you care for people over 65; or you live with or care for people of any age with chronic conditions.

- **Pneumococcus:** Vaccination is recommended if you are 65 or older or you have a serious health problem such as heart disease, sickle-cell disease, alcoholism, lung disease, diabetes, or **cirrhosis** of the liver.

- **Tetanus (lockjaw):** You should get a vaccinated if you have not had a booster shot in 10 years or more. If you never had the initial tetanus vaccines, you should get the series of three tetanus shots.

While these are the most common vaccines for adults, there are a number of others that adults may wish to consider. Following is a list of other diseases that are preventable with vaccines. The CDC recommends adults consult with their health-care provider about getting vaccinated for:

- haemophilus influenzae type b (Hib)
- hepatitis A
- hepatitis B
- herpes zoster (shingles)

- human papillomavirus (HPV)
- measles
- meningococcus
- mumps
- pertussis (whooping cough)
- polio
- rubella (German measles)
- varicella (chicken pox)

*See also:* Centers for Disease Control and Prevention (CDC); Epidemics and Pandemics; Infections, Bacterial and Viral; Influenza; Measles; Treatment

**FURTHER READING**
Bauman, Robert. *Microbiology.* San Francisco: Pearson, 2002.
Emmeluth, Donald. *Influenza.* Philadelphia: Chelsea House, 2003.
Shmaefsky, Brian R. *Meningitis.* Philadelphia: Chelsea House, 2005.


# ■ INFECTIONS, BACTERIAL AND VIRAL

Illnesses caused by microscopic **pathogens,** or disease agents. Pathogens causing **infectious** disease, from smallest to largest, include **viruses, bacteria, fungi, protists,** and **parasitic worms.** Pathogens are everywhere, and usually humans' natural defenses protect them from serious disease.

## THE IMMUNE SYSTEM'S RESPONSE TO PATHOGENS

The **immune system** provides physical and chemical barriers to infection. Skin and mucous membranes are the physical barriers that block invasion from most pathogens. If harmful pathogens get through these barriers, they trigger a second line of defense. Once inside the victim, the pathogen is known as an **antigen.** Antigens (usually viruses or bacteria) trigger the sending out of **antibodies,** which are proteins that attack and neutralize the pathogens. The antibodies, made to match the antigen, latch onto the pathogen and render it harmless or destroy it. Once the body has been invaded, large amounts of antibodies are made in glands under the arms or in the tonsils, which is why lumps in the armpits or sore throats are symptoms of some diseases. The glands are pouring large amounts of antibodies into the bloodstream to fight the infection. Once the pathogens get inside the cells, antibodies have no effect.

**Immunity** develops when the body has made antibodies against an antigen and thereafter "remembers" the antigen. The antibodies stay in the bloodstream, and if the antigen tries to invade again, antibodies can neutralize it before symptoms of the illness can occur.

## Immunization

Immunization is artificially building resistance to a disease without actually contracting it. Because of the antibody memory of the immune system, **vaccines,** or weakened or milder forms of a pathogen, trigger the production of antibodies without causing any symptoms. This gives immunity against the normal forms of the pathogens.

Another method of building up antibodies is by using a "killed" vaccine, or one in which the pathogens have been destroyed with a chemical. Then, even though the pathogen is inactive, the immune system still recognizes it and produces antibodies.

Humans can acquire immediate, temporary immunity, called passive immunity. In passive immunity, the person being immunized is not involved in making antibodies. An animal such as a horse is immunized, and makes antibodies that are collected from its blood and purified before being injected into humans. Another method of passive immunity is antibodies transferring from a mother to a fetus through the placenta, or through breast milk. Some vaccines give life-long protection, but others have to be repeated to remain effective.

## Cell-Mediated Immunity

**Cell-mediated immunity** occurs when various kinds of white blood cells fight pathogens. Most effective against cancer cells, **parasites,** and fungi, the cells recognize surface changes on body cells infected with pathogens and then bind to and kill the infected cells.

## VIRUSES

The smallest pathogens, viruses are parasites that depend on their hosts for all their needs. Basically, viruses are a set of instructions for making more viruses surrounded by a protective case. When a host develops an immunity, or resistance, to a virus, the host can become a **reservoir host,** in which the virus causes milder effects. For some human viruses, such as measles, humans are the reservoir hosts because different people have different levels of resistance to measles.

Viruses cause a number of diseases in humans, including those described below.

## AIDS
Acquired immunodeficiency syndrome is caused by the human immunodeficiency virus (HIV). HIV infects white blood cells and turns them into virus producers. During this process, the cells die, depriving the body of one of its defenses.

## Rabies
The virus is transmitted to humans through the infected saliva of rabid animals; it affects the central nervous system, the brain, and the spinal cord, and is fatal without treatment.

## Influenza
The flu virus spreads in droplets sprayed into the air by coughs and sneezes. New strains caused by mutations and by **gene swapping** can lead to epidemics, as humans have no resistance to the new forms of flu.

## Smallpox
The smallpox virus has caused repeated pandemics throughout history. The World Health Organization (WHO) initiated a program in 1967 that included **vaccination** and **quarantine.** In 1980, WHO announced that smallpox had been eliminated from the world, with the last known case reported in 1978. Isolated laboratory accidents now cause the only smallpox deaths.

## Ebola
Ebola is a viral infection passed between persons by direct contact with infected blood, body secretions, or organs. The mortality rate for Ebola infection is 90 percent. Ebola first appeared in 1976, when it caused 400 deaths in Zaire and Sudan in Africa. Several outbreaks have occurred since then.

## Measles
A highly contagious disease spread in airborne droplets and whose main symptom is a rash. Most contagious before the rash appears, the greatest risk of measles is in complications associated with the disease, which include pneumonia, inner ear infections, and, occasionally, encephalitis.

## Common Cold

Infection of the throat and nose caused by a virus. Usual symptoms include runny nose, sneezing, sore throat, coughing, and watery eyes. Colds spread through airborne droplets from coughs and sneezes and by touching objects that have been handled by a person with a cold.

## SARS

Originating in China in 2002, severe acute respiratory syndrome (SARS) is a viral disease that spread to 25 countries before it was contained in 2003. Symptoms of SARS are cough, difficulty breathing, fever, headache, body ache, and diarrhea. Eventually resulting in pneumonia, this disease spreads by close contact with an infected person. Although only eight people in the United States contracted the disease, 774 deaths resulted in the 8,100 people known to have the disease worldwide. Other than a few cases in China linked to laboratory research, no other cases had emerged through the summer of 2005.

## BACTERIAL DISEASES

Bacteria, at sizes of 40 to 800 millionths of an inch long, are much bigger than viruses. Bacteria that cause disease invade tissues or produce toxins (poisons). **Antibiotics,** drugs that kill or stop the growth of bacteria and fungi, are prescribed for treating bacterial diseases. Although patients may feel much better before a complete course of antibiotics is taken, the full course should be taken to ensure that all bacteria causing the illness are destroyed.

### Tuberculosis (TB)

The number one cause of death by a pathogen, TB kills between 2 million and 3 million people in the world each year; when an infected person coughs, the bacteria that cause TB are spread in droplets sprayed out. The droplets can remain in the air for two hours and still infect another person. Eating away at lung tissues until they no longer function, TB began to increase worldwide in the 1980s as new forms of the bacteria emerged. In 1998 the WHO warned that TB could infect 1 billion more people in the next 20 years and that 70 million of them are likely to die. A disease of the poor, TB most affects those who have the fewest physical and financial resources to combat it. Scientists continue to work on developing a drug effective against new strains of TB that are resistant to existing drugs.

### Cholera
Cholera is the most serious waterborne bacterial disease; the symptom of cholera is severe diarrhea that can result in the loss of five gallons of fluid per day and death by **dehydration.**

### Food Poisoning
Food poisoning is caused by eating food with bacterial toxins made by bacteria in food or by growth in the body of the bacteria that contaminated the food. Common sources are unrefrigerated dairy products, warm meat, contaminants on food from the animal itself or food handlers, and improper cooking. The main symptom is severe diarrhea followed by dehydration. Food poisoning is a major cause of death in underdeveloped countries and ranks second to the common cold as a cause of lost work time in developed countries. It is the fifth-leading cause of death in young children worldwide and can be life-threatening in the elderly.

## FUNGAL INFECTIONS
Fungi grow on moist parts of the body and can cause disease by producing an allergic reaction, by producing poisons, and by growing in or on the body. A normally healthy person's immune system is powerful enough to prevent invasion by nearly all fungi. An example of one of the most common fungal infections is athlete's foot, which can result from contact with infected lesions or by contact with contaminated shoes, towels, animals, or soil. Warm weather, humidity, and tight clothing encourage fungal growth. Topical antifungals are usually prescribed.

## PROTIST INFECTIONS
Protists are unicellular microorganisms, some of which cause deadly diseases. One of these, *Plasmodium,* causes malaria, which kills 2.7 million people a year, mostly children under five. About one-third of the world's population lives in areas with malaria, and at any one time, up to 500 million people are infected. If it is infected with *Plasmodia,* the female *Anopheles* mosquito injects saliva with thousands of parasites into the human bloodstream. In half an hour the parasites are inside liver cells, giving antibodies no time to kill them all. In two weeks, the liver cells burst and release large numbers of spores into the bloodstream. The sufferer then feels weak, tired, feverish, and suffers aches and pains. Ultimately, the parasite could invade 70 percent of the victim's red blood cells.

One challenge facing scientists trying to find a vaccine to treat malaria is that the parasite goes through four stages of development once inside a human. It is difficult to find a vaccine that would be effective against all four stages of the parasite's life while inside the host. Scientists are trying to develop vaccines by radiating infected mosquitoes and using **gene therapy**, but a vaccine is not in the immediate future.

### INFECTIONS BY PARASITIC WORMS

Helminths, including many types of parasitic worms, are the largest and most complex of the infectious disease agents. Roundworms (*Ascaris* worms) are probably the most common parasite in the world. Transmission to humans is caused by directly eating soil contaminated by human stool that has roundworm eggs or by eating poorly washed raw vegetables grown in contaminated soil. Symptoms include abdominal pain and lack of weight gain in children.

Tapeworms are usually caused by eating undercooked pork containing the larvae of the parasite. Once inside the human intestine, the larvae develop into adult worms, which can grow to lengths of 10 to 33 feet. Eggs leave the body in human feces. If pigs eat the feces, the parasite's life cycle continues. Sometimes in rural parts of Latin America people inadvertently eat the eggs, which then infect the central nervous system (brain and spinal cord) causing seizures and other disorders.

Hookworm disease is an infection of the upper intestine whose main symptom is anemia. The parasites live in sandy soil, with high humidity and a warm climate. Going barefoot in soil promotes transmission. This disease affects one-fourth the world's population and is seldom fatal.

*See also:* AIDS; Centers for Disease Control and Prevention (CDC); Epidemics and Pandemics; Immunization; Influenza; Measles; Sexually Transmitted Diseases (STDs); Skin Disorders; Strep Infections; Treatment

**FURTHER READING**
Snedden, Robert. *Fighting Infectious Diseases*. Chicago: Heinemann Library, 2007.

## ▪ INFLUENZA

A highly **contagious respiratory** illness caused by influenza **viruses**. Often called the flu, influenza has symptoms similar to those of the common cold and infects the nose, throat, and lungs. Unlike the common cold, influenza can cause severe illness with life-threatening complications for some people.

The many strains of influenza are grouped into three main types—A, B, and C. Type A strains cause frequent epidemics; types B and C are less common. Periodically, a type A strain of influenza will cause a pandemic.

### SYMPTOMS OF FLU

Symptoms of flu include fever (usually high), headache, extreme tiredness, dry cough, sore throat, runny or stuffy nose, muscle aches, nausea, vomiting, and diarrhea (usually in children).

### TRANSMISSION

When an infected person coughs or sneezes, the influenza virus in the respiratory droplets spreads from person to person. It is possible for people to spread the virus before they realize they are ill. Generally, adults are **infectious** for one day before the symptoms start until about five days after becoming sick. Research shows that children spread more influenza viruses for even longer periods of time. Another way people may become infected is by touching something with flu viruses on it and then touching their mouth or nose.

### PREVALENCE

CDC data show that, on average, 5 to 20 percent of the U.S. population gets the flu every year. In addition, more than 200,000 people are hospitalized from flu complications each year. Children under five years of age are hospitalized due to influenza complications as often as older people. About 36,000 people, mostly people over 65 years of age, die from the disease every year.

## Fact Or Fiction?

### If my symptoms are nausea, vomiting, and diarrhea, I have the flu.

**The Facts:** Symptoms of nausea, vomiting, and diarrhea are not really the flu, or influenza. The flu is a respiratory illness and high fever, cough, and overwhelming tiredness are often the key symptoms. Although someone might have some mild gastrointestinal symptoms, they are not usually the primary symptoms of flu. Most likely gastrointestinal symptoms mean you have viral gastroenteritis (a virus that is passed along from person to person that produces those symptoms) or food poisoning. Experts predict there are many more cases of mild to moderate food poisoning than we think because most people attribute them to "the flu" and don't seek medical care.

## COMPLICATIONS OF FLU

Older adults and young children are at high risk for flu complications; they are priority groups for getting the **vaccine** because they are less able to fight flu successfully on their own. Those complications can include **bacterial pneumonia,** ear infections, sinus infections, and **dehydration. Chronic** conditions such as asthma, diabetes, and heart disease can worsen when flu is contracted.

## PREVENTION

The Centers for Disease Control and Prevention (CDC) recommends yearly flu **vaccinations** for seasonal flu prevention. There are two types of vaccines. The flu shot contains an inactivated vaccine, which contains a killed virus. The nasal-spray flu vaccine contains live, weakened flu viruses that do not cause flu. Researchers had wanted to develop a less invasive way than a needle to give the vaccine, but a live virus must be used. Because people with suppressed **immune systems** could be susceptible to even a weak form of a live virus, they would get very ill if they should develop the flu, and they are not usually given the live-virus vaccines.

### Who Should Get the Influenza Vaccination?

Vaccinations are available for all people who want to reduce their chances of getting the flu. Those people who are at high risk of having flu-related complications or people who live with those at high risk are advised to get vaccinated each year. The CDC's Advisory Committee on Immunization Practices (ACIP) defines the priority groups for vaccination when vaccine supplies are limited during flu seasons. The highest priority group contains people at high risk for complications from the flu. These include:

- children aged six months to five years
- pregnant women
- people 50 years of age and older
- people of any age with certain chronic medical conditions

- people who live in nursing homes and other long-term care facilities

The next highest priority group contains those who live with or care for people at high risk for complications from flu, including:

- household contacts of persons at high risk for complications from flu
- household contacts and out-of-home caregivers of children less than 6 months of age
- health-care workers

On the bottom of the priority list are the rest of the general population, who may wish to decrease their risk of influenza.

Healthy People 2010, a government-sponsored initiative designed to improve the health of people in the United States, identifies as one of its goals having 90 percent of people 65 and older receive annual influenza vaccinations by the year 2010. Immunization rates in older adults have risen from 33 percent in 1989 to 64 percent in 1998.

### Who Should Use the Nasal-Spray Flu Vaccine?

Healthy people of two to 49 years of age who are not pregnant, and even healthy people living with or caring for those in the high-risk group, can use the nasal-spray flu vaccine. An exception is healthy people who care for those with severely weakened immune systems who require a protected environment—those caretakers should get the flu shot (inactivated vaccine) so that there is no chance of the caretaker acting as a flu **carrier** to those with weak immune systems.

# Fact Or Fiction?

*The influenza vaccine doesn't work.*

**The Facts:** The influenza vaccine prevents the flu in 77 to 91 percent of children and teens (children one to 16 years old). If someone gets the flu after getting vaccinated, he or she may have been exposed to the influenza virus before the vaccination or before the vaccine had taken effect. Usually, these people get a milder case of influenza. Also, it can take up to two weeks for the body to develop protective **antibodies** against the flu. During that time, there is still a risk of getting sick.

## Who Should Not Be Vaccinated?

A health-care provider should be consulted before these people are vaccinated:

- people with severe allergies to chicken eggs—the vaccine contains egg protein, and viruses that are used to make the vaccine are grown in eggs, so a quantity of the chicken-egg allergen could still be present and the person could have a severe allergic reaction

- people who have reacted severely to influenza vaccinations in the past—they may have a severe reaction again

- people who have developed Guillain-Barré syndrome (GBS) within six weeks of a past flu vaccination—GBS is a severe disease and another episode cannot be risked

- children under six months old—their immune systems are too undeveloped to resist the risk of the weakened or killed virus

- people with moderate or severe illnesses with fevers—they should wait until symptoms lessen; they will not form adequate antibodies to the vaccine, because their bodies are already fighting illnesses

## Everyday Preventive Actions

Everyday precautions can reduce your risk of getting and spreading the flu, such as covering your nose and mouth with a tissue when you cough or sneeze and then throwing away the used tissue. You should wash your hands often with soap and water, especially when you cough and sneeze. Use an alcohol-based hand cleanser if you are not near water. As much as possible, try to avoid sick people, and stay home if you get the flu so that you do not spread the virus. Avoid touching your eyes, nose, or mouth.

## Antiviral Drugs

If you develop flu symptoms or are exposed to the flu before getting vaccinated, your health-care provider can prescribe antiviral drugs if appropriate. The antiviral drugs that can treat the flu should be started within 48 hours of getting sick. For prevention, the drugs are 70 to 90 percent effective for shortening the time of illness and reducing the severity of the illness. If the drugs are not taken in the very short window of getting the illness, they are ineffective.

## IF YOU GET THE FLU

Most healthy people recover from the flu without complications. The CDC recommends that if you get the flu, you should stay home, rest, drink fluids, and avoid alcohol and tobacco. There are over-the-counter(OTC) medications that will relieve flu symptoms. Children and teens should never take aspirin if they have fevers and flu-like symptoms. If you are in a high-risk group, you should take into account the risk of complications, and be aware of warning signs that the illness is becoming abnormally severe or even life-threatening.

In children, these warning signs indicate urgent medical attention is needed: fast or troubled breathing, bluish skin color, dehydration, non-responsiveness, irritability, not wanting to be held, lessening of symptoms followed by a return of fever and a worse cough, and a fever with rash.

In adults, these are the warning signs indicating the need for urgent medical attention: difficulty breathing, shortness of breath, chest or abdominal pain or pressure, sudden dizziness, confusion, and severe or persistent vomiting.

## THE SPANISH FLU OF 1918

Infecting 20 to 40 percent of the world's population between September 1918 and April 1919, the Spanish flu killed more than 20 million people worldwide. In the United States, about 500,000 people died. Attacking young and old, the Spanish flu could strike and kill a person in one day. Even if people survived the initial illness, they could develop pneumonia and die days or weeks later. Health-care providers often fell victim to the illness as they were infected treating others. In the spring of 1919, the epidemic faded and did not return.

Although the Spanish flu was an unusually severe influenza pandemic, other epidemics followed. The Asian flu epidemic (1957–58), and two epidemics of the Hong Kong flu (1968–69; 1970–72) resulted from influenza spreading among people lacking immunity to a new strain of virus. With increasing globalization and increasingly accessible airline travel, a new strain could travel the world in a short time. An example of a worldwide flu scare is the Severe Acute Respiratory Syndrome (SARS) outbreak of 2003.

## SARS

SARS is a viral respiratory illness that started in Asia in February of 2003. Over the next few months, the illness spread to two dozen countries in North America, South America, Europe, and Asia, before the global outbreak was contained. According to the World Health Organization, 8,096 people became sick with SARS and 774 died. Spread by person-to-person contact, the disease ws transmitted by travelers from Asia. In the United States, 800 medical experts at the CDC responded to the outbreak. Once the problem was identified, information and alerts were sent to the world, and all people flying out of China were screened to successfully contain the disease.

## H1N1 FLU (SWINE FLU)

In April 2009, in the same way that seasonal flu spreads, H1N1 flu began spreading in the United States from person to person. Three months later, a pandemic was declared by the World Health Organization, when 74 countries reported 27,737 cases and 141 deaths. Originally called swine flu, many of the virus's genes were thought to be similar to viruses in North American pigs. People with H1N1 flu not only experience symptoms similar to seasonal flu, but some who get the virus also experience diarrhea and vomiting. The same people at high risk for serious complications from seasonal flu are at high risk for severe illnesses and death as a result of this virus.

*See also:* Allergies; Centers for Disease Control and Prevention (CDC); Epidemics and Pandemics; Immunization; Infections, Bacterial and Viral

**FURTHER READING**
DeSalle, Rob, ed. *Epidemic! The World of Infectious Disease.* New York: New Press and American Museum of Natural History, 1999.
Emmeluth, Donald. *Influenza.* Philadelphia: Chelsea House, 2003.
Ward, Brian. *Epidemic.* New York: Dorling Kindersley, 2000.

# ■ LEUKEMIA

Cancer of the blood and bone marrow. Leukemia begins in a cell in the bone marrow, which produces all blood cells. The cell changes and replicates itself many times. These leukemia cells grow and crowd out the normal blood cells in the blood and bone marrow.

In **acute,** or sudden onset, leukemia, there is too high or too low a number of immature white blood cells. The original leukemia cell can form a trillion more leukemia cells. White blood cells in some **chronic** forms of leukemia look as though they have matured but have not; they live longer than they should, build up, and cause problems.

## CAUSES AND RISKS

Some types of leukemia affect adults, and several types affect children. The exact cause of leukemia is unknown, but scientists have identified some likely contributing factors. Some leukemia cases are thought to be affected by prolonged exposure to radiation, certain chemicals, **viruses,** genetic abnormalities, and chronic exposure to benzene.

## SYMPTOMS

Many symptoms of leukemia are similar to those of other illnesses. Diagnosis can be confirmed with blood tests and bone marrow tests. Symptoms may include tiredness and lack of energy, shortness of breath during activity, mild fever, excess bleeding and slow healing of cuts, bruises, red spots under the skin, aches in bones and **joints,** and low white blood cell counts.

## COPING AND TREATMENT

Complete **remission** is the goal of leukemia treatment. Remission of leukemia means a return to normal white blood cell levels and normal functioning of those cells. Increasingly, leukemia patients in the United States are in complete remission at five years following treatment. Many patients begin **chemotherapy** and drug treatment immediately after their diagnosis. Leukemia was the first type of cancer that was treated with chemotherapy. It may not cure the cancer, but chemo may keep the cancer under control for a long time. Side effects of the chemo are hair loss, vomiting, loss of appetite, tiredness, nausea, and diarrhea. Because some developing blood cells can be killed along with the cancer cells, anemia can develop, which is treated with blood transfusions. People's reactions to chemotherapy vary, and continuing normal activities is dependent on the side effects.

Bone marrow (stem cell) transplants may be used. When blood cells are made in the bone marrow they start out as stem cells, which grow and turn into the different blood cell types that make up the blood. A bone marrow transplant allows new stem cells to start growing and becoming healthy mature cells.

People with leukemia need to exercise, eat right, get enough sleep, avoid stress, try to stay positive about the treatment process, accept help and support from friends and family, and learn as much as possible about the disease.

# TEENS SPEAK

## Tyler Has Leukemia

My name is Tyler, and I was diagnosed with leukemia last year. I have AML—acute myelogenous leukemia. I'm 16. I was starting baseball practice in the spring and got hit with a ball. Hey, it happens, no big deal. But four weeks later my mom noticed I still had this horrible bruise and I had not been acting like myself. Truth is, I wasn't feeling good at all, but I love baseball season and wanted to make the varsity squad, so I was trying to get through it all. My schoolwork was falling off because I'd come home after practice and go to sleep.

When my mom saw the big bruise there, she insisted I go to the doctor, and he did a very thorough evaluation. He talked about how pale I looked, and mom and I had noticed that, too. He asked about the many bruises I had, and I noticed they were all over—like nothing I had ever seen from playing sports. I was hurting, too. It felt like it hurt right down to my bones, and my weight had dropped down. So when the doctor suggested getting some lab tests I really did not protest since I just wanted to feel better.

My parents were both home that night when the doctor called them and told them he thought I might have leukemia. The blood tests he did showed I had a very abnormal blood count that went along with what he saw on my exam. I didn't even know what leukemia was. I found out it was a cancer of the blood-forming cells. I still can't believe it some days.

I was sent to a doctor specializing in kids with leukemia and had a million more tests done. A bone marrow biopsy was done by taking a sample from my hip area in the bone; it was a lot of pressure and felt very uncomfortable. I also had a lymph node biopsy where they took a lymph node out to examine it. Because cancer in the blood has easy access to the whole body, it was important to find out how much it had spread. A bunch more labs were taken and I had X-rays, CT scans, and MRIs.

They ended up hospitalizing me because I got an infection and needed IV antibiotics. I learned this is common because my white blood cells are not very good—they don't fight infection like they should. Once the infection was treated they had figured out my protocol. A protocol comes from the National Cancer Institute and analyzes my data to look at the best possible treatment options. Then the doctors and nurses started treating my cancer.

I am lucky I guess. I live near a children's cancer center where this has to be treated. Some other kids in there have to come four and five hours to get here, and their parents are stuck going back and forth and figuring out how to work. My parents can go home at night to sleep and take turns for who is with me and who watches my sister.

At the first phase of my chemotherapy the treatment cycles last for several days at a time, and I have to do it again every two weeks. It took three treatments before the bone marrow showed no leukemia. I also got chemo into the spinal column—that was weird but not really painful. That was the first part.

The next part started once the bone marrow was clear. I got high-dose chemo for months, and I just ended it this month. During this time I also had three blood transfusions and I don't know how many antibiotics for infections. I used to love to eat, but now it's a chore to eat. Mom and the nurses are always reminding me that it's important to keep my strength up because it will help me fight infection.

If all goes well, I have a 75 to 85 percent chance of remission. Right now the team is all keeping a close eye on me with labs and exams and watching my temperature. I'll have more tests again soon to look at the bone marrow and the rest of my body.

If I don't go into and stay in remission, then we may talk about a stem cell transplant. It would probably have to come from my sister, who is only 14, so I hope we don't have to do that. However, I know my chances for a long-term cure would be better if I did have a stem cell transplant.

I'm just beginning to think about the emotional impact of this on me and my family. They have been so great, and everything else going on in the family just stopped while they focused on me and my treatment. But I'm 16, and I want to be out with my friends and dating and driving a car—not sitting on a couch too tired to walk around the block. I'm trying to be positive and think about maybe playing baseball next year (do NOT tell my parents). The doctors and nurses have been outstanding, and I am thinking about a career in something medical now. For today I'm just going to think about staying healthy.

*See also:* Cancer; Treatment

**FURTHER READING**
Apel, Melanie Ann. *Coping with Leukemia.* New York: Rosen, 2001.

# ■ LUNG DISEASE
*See*: Immunization

# ■ LYME DISEASE
An **infection** caused by type of **bacteria** passed to humans by ticks. According to the Center for Disease Control and Prevention (CDC), ticks carrying the bacteria are most commonly found in the northeastern United States. Lyme disease has been reported in every state but Montana. New York, New Jersey, Pennsylvania, and Connecticut report the highest numbers of cases. The highest rates of Lyme disease are found in south-central Connecticut, Westchester County and Eastern Long Island in New York, the southern coast of New Jersey, and Cape Cod and Nantucket in Massachusetts. Other states with high rates are California, Minnesota, and Wisconsin. Connecticut's incidence rate is double that of every other state.

More than 145,000 cases have been reported since 1982, which makes it the most common disease in the United States that is spread by a vector. A **vector** is a living thing or object that passes along a disease but is not itself affected by the disease. In 2007, the CDC estimates the incidence of Lyme disease as 9.1 cases per 100,000 people in the United States.

## DID YOU KNOW?

# Protecting Yourself from Lyme Disease

While enjoying the pleasures and benefits of hiking, gardening, camping, fishing, and other outdoor activities, especially if you live in or vacation in prime habitats for deer ticks, the American Lyme Disease Foundation recommends you take these precautions:

- Wear light-colored clothes that are tightly woven.
- Always wear enclosed shoes or boots.
- Wear long pants tucked into your socks and a long-sleeved shirt tucked into your pants.
- Before going into the woods, spray your clothes with insect repellent.
- Wear a hat; pull hair back so that it doesn't touch long grass or bushes.
- When gardening, pruning, or picking up dead leaves, wear light-colored gloves and check frequently for ticks.
- Avoid sitting on the ground or on stone walls where small animals like mice and chipmunks, which often carry ticks, may hide. If you attend a concert or picnic on the ground, sit on an insect repellant-sprayed blanket or a lawn chair.
- Hike on clear, well-traveled paths.
- In the woods or garden, check for ticks every three to four hours.
- Change clothes right away after hiking or fishing. Remove outer clothing layers away from the living area of the house. Check clothes for ticks and wash them as soon as possible.
- Shower and wash your hair; check your entire body for ticks as soon as you get home.

Ticks are active when the temperature is above 40°F. A complete self-examination whenever you are outside in a woody or grassy area is the best protection against infection.

Source: American Lyme Disease Foundation, 2004.

## TRANSMISSION

Ticks, mice, and deer carry bacteria called *Borrelia burgdorferi*. When a tick carrying the bacteria bites a person, it infects the bloodstream with the bacteria, which travels throughout the body. The bacteria can attack the **joints** and nervous system.

## STAGE I SYMPTOMS

Usually, one to two weeks after being bitten, the first symptom of Lyme disease appears. It is an expanding skin rash that is lighter in the center at the site of the bite with darker, red rings surrounding it. It greatly resembles a bull's-eye. The bloodstream already has the bacteria in it, and they may already have reached the spinal fluid by this time. A slight fever, mild headache, and general aches may accompany the rash.

Unfortunately, the rash does not appear in 30 to 40 percent of Lyme disease cases. If people do not see the rash, they may assume their symptoms indicate that they have the flu and may lose valuable time in treating the disease, allowing it to progress to later stages.

## STAGE II SYMPTOMS

Weeks or months after the bacterial infection, if left untreated, more symptoms appear. In children, painful, swollen joints, a kind of arthritis, are a sign that the Lyme disease is in stage II. In children, more than 90 percent of the time, knees are affected by Lyme arthritis. The arthritis can progress very quickly, causing inability to walk in 24 hours.

As the disease affects the nervous system, a stiff neck and severe headaches can also appear. Paralyzed facial muscles may cause one side of the face to droop, a condition known as Bell's palsy. Adults may have a variety of symptoms other than these. In fact, Lyme disease is called "the great imitator" because it causes symptoms very similar to other diseases such as multiple sclerosis, **infectious** mononucleosis, and chronic fatigue syndrome. This makes the disease difficult to diagnose, and health-care providers need to know about any outdoor trips or events that could have been the site of ticks.

## TREATMENT

Lyme disease is almost always cured by **antibiotics** if treatment starts within three to six weeks of the day of infection. The key is early treatment before the disease reaches stage II and spreads. If the disease reaches stage II, intravenous antibiotics and hospitalization will be required.

*See also:* Infections, Bacterial and Viral

**FURTHER READING**
Donnelly, Karen. *Coping with Lyme Disease.* New York: Rosen, 2001.
Yannielli, Len. *Lyme Disease.* Philadelphia: Chelsea House, 2004.

# ■ MEASLES

A **respiratory** infection caused by a highly **contagious virus.** Worldwide, 30 to 40 million cases of measles occur every year, resulting in 1 million deaths. A red rash, high fever, runny nose, cough, sore throat, and white spots in the mouth are symptoms. Spreading easily through airborne droplets, measles is most contagious before the rash occurs.

By the fifth day of infection, the symptoms diminish; immunity to further measles infection is then permanent. Treatment for the measles includes bed rest and fever-reducing medicines—but not aspirin. Potentially, the measles can set one up for pneumonia, seizures related to high fevers, or death.

## PREVALENCE

Before 1963, when the **vaccine** became available in the United States, 3 to 4 million cases of measles occurred in the U.S. annually. Measles killed 400 to 500 children a year and put 48,000 in the hospital. Due to the measles vaccine, fewer than 50 cases of measles occurred in the United States in 2004. But, by spring 2008, outbreaks of measles had been reported in seven states, and the total cases for the year were predicted to be higher than in any other recent year. The largest outbreaks were caused by international travelers spreading the disease to unvaccinated people. Worldwide, 18 million children get measles each year and 242,000 children die from it. Efforts to increase **vaccinations** are being made. The Measles Initiative, a partnership of the American Red Cross, Centers for Disease Control and Prevention (CDC), the United Nations Foundation, UNICEF, and the World Health Organization seeks to reduce the number of deaths due to measles by 90 percent worldwide by 2010.

## PREVENTION

Vaccination for measles is given in conjunction with mumps, rubella, and varicella (the MMRV vaccine) and the vaccine is approved for children aged 12 months through 12 years of age (and up to age 13). The composition of the measles vaccine is a live virus and is 95 percent effective; the duration of the immunity is lifelong and includes a schedule of two doses. The vaccine can fail in a person who has had measles, mumps, or rubella previously (lacked immunity). Two to 5 percent of those vaccinated do not respond to the first dose; errors can be caused by antibodies, a damaged vaccine, or record errors. Most people in whom the first dose fails will respond to the second dose.

# Q & A

## Question: What Is "German" Measles?

**Answer:** German measles, or rubella, is a mildly contagious disease caused by a virus. Since a vaccine against it was introduced in 1969, no epidemics have occurred, and in 2005, the CDC determined that rubella was eradicated in the United States. Still, the CDC recommends that vaccination be continued because the virus can be introduced by travelers from abroad.

*See also:* Centers for Disease Control and Prevention (CDC); Epidemics and Pandemics; Immunization

**FURTHER READING**

The Mayo Clinic. "Measles." URL: www.mayoclinic.com/health/measles/DS00331. Accessed February 12, 2009.

The Measles Initiative. "Measles." URL: www.measlesinitiative.org/index3.asp. Accessed July 17, 2008.

# ■ MIGRAINE HEADACHE

Episodes of head pain accompanied by nausea, vomiting, and sensitivity to light and sound. Twenty-eight million Americans experience the severe pain of migraine, and 75 percent of them are women. Migraines have a significant effect on work and school life because patients often experience them one to two times a month, or more.

Because the pain gets worse when the patient moves about, especially when there are lights and sound, it can be difficult to perform normal activities. Part of the treatment is resting in a quiet, dark room. The age of onset is usually between 10 and 46 years; it is rare to have a new onset after age 50.

## DID YOU KNOW?

# Migraines and Gender

A higher percentage of women than men experience severe headaches or migraines.

- 20.8 percent of females suffer from severe headaches or migraines.

- 9.7 percent of males suffer from severe headaches or migraines.

Source: Centers for Disease Control and Prevention, National Center for Health Statistics, National Health Interview Survey, 2007.

## SYMPTOMS

Migraines generally follow a pattern. One of the most important diagnostic tools is tracking the history, patterns, and symptoms of the headaches. The symptoms of most migraine headaches, called classic migraines, include worse pain on one side of the head than the other; pounding or throbbing pain of moderate to severe intensity; and an increase in the pain due to activity. Nausea, vomiting, and sensitivity to light and/or noises are also typical.

### Classic Migraine with Aura

An aura is a visual disturbance of less than 60 minutes that usually signals the coming of a migraine. The symptoms of an aura develop gradually, in about five minutes, and they stop entirely between attacks. About 30 percent of people who get migraines experience auras. A person experiencing an aura may see flashing lights, spots, stars, color splashes, or waves that shimmer or flicker. Other aura characteristics are numbing or tingling of skin, muscle weakness, and problems using or understanding language. Sometimes a person experiences the aura but the actual migraine headache never develops. A classic migraine can last from several minutes to one to two days.

### Common Migraine without Aura

Migraine without aura is more common than those with auras. Although no universal warning signs foretell the coming of common migraine, some people claim mood changes or loss of appetite occur before attacks. The nature of a person's headaches can change over a lifetime, evolving from one type to another.

## STAGES OF MIGRAINES

Most people experience more than one phase of a migraine attack.

Premonitory phase: Not an aura, premonitory symptoms can go unnoticed or be experienced as "just a bad day." Common symptoms are **depression**, fatigue or weakness, difficulty concentrating, and a stiff neck.

Aura phase: Aura sensations may be mild or intense, and may vary among attacks. Usually occurring 20 minutes before an attack, most auras last 10 to 25 minutes. Some examples of auras are flashing lights in the vision, zigzag patterns in the vision, or blind spots. Some may be even more dramatic.

Headache: This includes throbbing head pain, moderate to severe in intensity, becoming worse with increased activity. In 60 percent of attacks the pain is on one side of the head; in the remaining 40 percent pain is on both sides. Usually starting in the morning, the aching builds up over minutes or hours. Some people are disabled, but most people suffer less than a day. In addition to the head pain, nausea, intolerance to light, sensitivity to noise, and aversion to odors can occur. An attack can be accompanied by paleness of skin, chills, sweating, clammy hands and feet, and weight gain from fluid retention. Sufferers can also experience gastrointestinal problems; swelling of the scalp or face; bulging blood vessels in the temple; stiff neck; difficulty concentrating and thinking clearly; feelings of depression, fatigue, **anxiety**, and irritability; and lightheadedness.

Post-headache phase: During this phase, all signs and symptoms disappear. Sleep or vomiting can end the attack followed by a range of feelings from depression to elation.

## MIGRAINE TRIGGERS

Many people with migraines find that attacks occur in response to specific events or situations, such as eating certain foods, encountering strong odors, and experiencing weather changes or stress. Migraines can result from skipping meals, dieting, fasting, and missing usual daily caffeine. Too much or too little sleep, physical activity, hormonal changes, visual and auditory triggers, motion sickness, environmental factors, prescription medications, neck pain, and medical conditions can all trigger migraines as well.

## CAUSES

Migraines occur when the brain's neural pathways register pain even though there is no external source for the pain. Some scientists theorize chemical imbalances in the brain cause migraines; others think there is a disorder in the way some people's brains and blood vessels work, making them more susceptible to headaches. One theory is that, instead of moving along a nerve smoothly, impulses become jumbled and end up at blood vessels in the brain's protective covering and in the scalp. These blood vessels relax, fill with blood, and become inflamed. Nerve endings in the brain and scalp are activated and send a message of pain to the brain resulting in a headache.

The female hormone estrogen is also connected to migraines and may be the reason many more women than men have migraines. This may also be the reason so many women have migraines around the time of their periods, when estrogen levels change.

Researchers have long known there is a connection between **genetics** and migraines. More than 60 percent of people suffering from migraines have close relatives who also get them. Scientists are conducting research to pinpoint the exact chromosome that may be responsible for migraines.

Another theory about the cause of migraines is based on the electrical activity of the brain. Normally, electrical charges in the brain cause the different areas of the body to function. One theory alleges that there may be an abnormal burst of electrical activity in the brain stimulating many different areas at one time—areas that normally are not stimulated at the same time—which leads to the migraine.

## TREATMENT

Treatment of migraines involves two major strategies: lifestyle management and drug therapy. Lifestyle management includes eating a healthful diet, getting plenty of sleep, getting enough exercise, avoiding stress, and modifying some behaviors, such as eating, sleeping, and relaxing. Additionally, discovering what triggers an individual's migraines and then avoiding those triggers if at all possible is a good method of prevention. Drugs are given for both **acute** (for rapid relief of pain) and preventive treatment of migraines.

### Nonsteroidal Anti-inflammatory Medications

Pain relieving medications should be taken as soon as the migraine patient suspects he or she has a migraine "coming on." Learning to be alert to auras and premonitory symptoms can be helpful in starting medication early. Some of the first medications used to treat migraines are nonsteroidal **anti-inflammatory** drugs (NSAIDs). These include aspirin and ibuprofen and can help relieve mild migraines.

### SEROTONIN BLOCKERS

Many people who have severe migraines need to use triptans, a group of medicines that more quickly and effectively relieve migraine pain. They work by blocking serotonin in the brain and short-circuiting the pain. Some are taken by pill and some can be taken by injection. Known for their quick relief of migraines, these drugs do have side effects as well, and some people notice a rapid heart rate shortly after taking them. Ergotamine has been used for many years, but its popularity has declined as it is less effective than the newer triptans. Occasionally, a migraine patient may use medication to treat nausea symptoms, but this is not common.

### PREVENTION

When a patient has several migraines per month, the health-care provider and patient often elect to try medications to prevent the migraine altogether. Some medications are beta blockers, tricyclic **antidepressants**, antiseizure medication, a specific **antihistamine** called cyprohepatadine, and Botox injections.

# TEENS SPEAK

## Coping with Migraines

My name is Karen. I'm 19 and away at college now, but I've had these migraine headaches for years. Now that I've learned a little and I look back, I can see I had them since I was about 12. One of the things I've been learning is what my triggers are. Triggers are the things that set off this kind of headache. For me, my hormonal shifts are the biggest trigger. Some people get them with certain food, like cheese, but I have never noticed that. My migraines can also be triggered by weather and stress.

Some people get warnings, or auras, and those can be kind of scary and strange. Some get flashing lights or blind spots in their vision. I only get tightness in my neck on the side I get the headache and it just gets worse over time until I realize my head is beginning to throb. The headache is usually located on one side of my head and feels like it sits right behind my eyes. Sometimes I get sick to my stomach, which I know is pretty common.

For years I didn't know these were different kinds of headaches and we really didn't think much of it at home. I have an older sister who has had bad headaches as long as I can remember and she took over-the-counter medicine like aspirin and just worked around it, so I thought that was just how I would be.

When I started college last year, the headaches became increasingly severe and they would affect my ability to study and take tests because I had such a throbbing sensation that I couldn't concentrate. One of my roommates ended up taking me to student health services when one got so bad that my vision blurred and I started vomiting. They did an MRI of my brain to make sure it wasn't a tumor and that turned out normal, so they tried some special migraine medication that's new in the last few years. Within 10 minutes I could sit up and my headache was completely gone. I was used to dealing with the pain and symptoms for a couple days before I would get better and this was such relief. They had me follow up with my doctor, and he had me do a "headache diary," which is basically a recording of when I have a headache, what's going on, and what I ate and drank beforehand. That way I could avoid the triggers I can control and be prepared with the proper medication when the headaches occur.

While I know I will have to deal with migraines for some time, at least I feel that I can treat them effectively now and I can study and go about my day once I treat them. I would encourage anyone who has severe headaches to see their health-care provider to get them checked out.

*See also:* Genetic Disorders

**FURTHER READING**

Swanson, Jerry W. *Mayo Clinic on Headache*. Rochester, Minn.: Mayo Foundation, 2004.

Votava, Andrea. *Coping with Migraines and Other Headaches*. New York: Rosen, 1997.

# ■ MONONUCLEOSIS, INFECTIOUS

An **infectious** disease caused by the Epstein-Barr **virus**. Commonly affecting teens and young adults, mononucleosis saps a person's energy and makes simple things such as brushing one's hair or carrying a backpack exhausting.

### SYMPTOMS AND TRANSMISSION OF MONO

Fatigue, fever, sore throat, and swollen lymph glands are symptoms of "mono." In addition, headaches, loss of appetite, skin rash, muscle aches, and an enlarged spleen are other possible symptoms. Mono is transferred among people through direct contact with saliva. Sharing a cup, food, eating utensil—anything that touches a person's mouth—can lead to mono.

One factor that makes it difficult to avoid the disease is that avoiding people with the disease does not ensure protection from it. A person may spread the virus without having symptoms of mono. In fact, people who are healthy and already immune to the disease are the most common means of spreading the disease.

---

**DID YOU KNOW?**

## Transmission of Mono

Although it is often referred to as "the kissing disease," there are many other ways to pass saliva between people and get mononucleosis. The virus can also be transmitted by the following:

- children sharing toys
- sharing lip gloss
- using someone else's straw
- passing around a water bottle at sports practice
- brushing with someone else's toothbrush
- playing another's musical instrument such as a trombone or a flute
- eating food from someone else's plate
- sharing eating utensils

Source: Mayo Clinic, 2008.

The Epstein-Barr virus has a 30–50 day incubation period when it multiplies and spreads inside the body. Because the infected person shows no symptoms during this time, the person can give the disease to someone else without knowing it.

A single type of virus, the Epstein-Barr virus, causes 90 percent of mononucleosis cases. A member of the herpesvirus family, the Epstein-Barr virus is a close relative of the viruses that cause cold sores and chicken pox. One of the most common viruses in the world, scientists estimate that the Epstein-Barr virus will infect more than 90 percent of the world's people at some time in their lives. Only a small number of those people infected will ever develop symptoms of mono.

### IMMUNITY

If a person develops **immunity** to the Epstein-Barr virus as a child, that immunity will protect the person from developing mono as a teen or adult when infected again with the virus. People can develop immunity when, as young children, they fight the infection without getting mono symptoms, or the symptoms are mild and are interpreted as a mild case of flu. However, the **antibodies** that build up against the virus stay in the body and help protect against infection later. If a person has first contact with the virus as a teen, though, he or she would not already have antibodies able to recognize and fight the virus, thus making him or her more likely to get sick. Teens are about 100 times more likely to develop mono symptoms than children younger than five.

### TREATMENT

The **acute** phase of mono—when you have the fever, sore throat, swollen lymph glands, and fatigue—usually lasts two weeks. At this time, you are most **contagious,** or most likely to spread the disease to others. About 50 percent of patients can return to school or work within two weeks, but mono can leave you feeling tired for a long time after the other symptoms have gone. It can take two to three months before you return to feeling normal.

It is not necessary to isolate mono patients, but it is necessary to avoid the exchange of saliva. Getting plenty of rest, drinking fluids, taking a nonaspirin pain reliever, and eating a balanced diet are normal treatments. Scientists are working on developing an Epstein-Barr **vaccine** that will cause immune cells to create antibodies.

# TEENS SPEAK

## *My Mono Diagnosis*

I'm Glen and I'm 15. I like to sleep in on weekends, but shortly after winter break last year, I felt like I could not get enough sleep. I'd sleep 12 hours a night on weekends and still be tired. I'd come home from school and go to sleep. At first I thought it was just classes (algebra!) and basketball practices and games.

Then one day I noticed my neck was really swollen and it looked like little golf balls in there. My mom made me go to the doctor, and he said I had swollen lymph glands and a fever. He also felt for my spleen under my left rib cage and said it was swollen. So the doctor did a blood test and confirmed that I had infectious mononucleosis ("mono").

The doctor told me mono is very common in young people and I had the classic signs and symptoms. He said it's often called the "kissing disease" because the mono is passed along in saliva but it's often passed by other ways, and I did share a water bottle at basketball practice one day. In fact, the kid that owned the bottle was out sick for awhile, too.

There is no cure but rest to let the body fight the infection. That's why the glands and spleen get big—the body tries to gear up for fighting the infection. Resting was hard because it meant I missed school for a couple of weeks, and I wasn't allowed to play basketball until my spleen size went down, because some ordinary basketball move could have ruptured the spleen. I didn't have energy to play anyway. I did my school assignments online to keep up.

Even when I went back to school, I had to take it easy—sitting out gym and basketball at first. After a month, I felt more like my old self and the doctor said I could go back to basketball and gym classes. Soon I was back to my usual routine.

*See also:* Infections, Bacterial and Viral; Treatment

**FURTHER READING**
Hoffmann, Gretchen. *Mononucleosis.* New York: Marshall Cavendish, 2006.

# ■ MULTIPLE SCLEROSIS

A nervous system disease that causes the muscles to weaken, twitch, or clench involuntarily. A **chronic** disease, it affects vision and sensation. Symptoms of multiple sclerosis (MS) can come and go; an attack caused by stress can bring the symptoms back or the symptoms can come back with no reason. Thus far, scientists are not certain what causes MS.

MS targets the myelin, or white matter, a fatty substance in a sheath insulating the brain and nervous system. During an MS attack, the myelin becomes inflamed, and the **inflammations** leave lesions on the brain and spinal cord, which become covered with scar tissue (sclerosis). Because there are many such lesions, the disease is called multiple sclerosis.

## WHO GETS MULTIPLE SCLEROSIS?

Adults between the ages of 20 and 40 account for the majority of cases. Twice as many women as men are affected, and the disease occurs earlier in women than in men. Caucasians almost exclusively develop the disease. People who grow up in temperate climates such as the United States, Canada, and most of Europe are at greater risk for getting MS (1 in 2,000) than people in tropical climates, such as Central America and Africa (1 in 10,000). Growing up near the equator lowers a person's risk even further.

## SYMPTOMS

Symptoms include continuous muscle contraction causing stiffness or tightness of muscles. Walking, movement, and speech may be affected. Involuntary twitching of muscles may occur. The person may experience an inability to maintain balance while walking and may feel a sensation of burning or prickling on skin for no apparent cause.

# Q & A

**Question: I've noticed that I've had some tremors and loss of balance lately—does this mean I have MS?**

**Answer:** For a reliable diagnosis, check with your health-care provider. For a diagnosis of MS, a person must have two flare-ups at least a month apart and a myelin sheath with more than one area of scarring on the brain. A test called **magnetic resonance imaging (MRI),** can reveal scarring of the myelin sheath on some areas, but much more information is needed for an accurate diagnosis.

## TYPES

There are a number of different types of MS. The mildest and most common in which patients have flare-ups lasting for days, weeks, or months followed by complete recovery; the disease does not progress between flare-ups. A second type includes progressive weakness between flares. These flares are seen as the patient ages. A third type is a steadily worsening form of MS with no **remission**; this type is seen in 10 percent of cases.

## COPING AND TREATMENT

Although there is no cure for MS, there are treatments for its symptoms. Though many are treated with medications, some people with MS do well with no drug therapy at all other than over-the-counter remedies such as **anti-inflammatories**. Some need medication only occasionally, during a flare-up. Some need partial or complete care by others and are wheelchair-bound.

*See also:* Chronic Disease

### FURTHER READING

Aaseng, Nathan. *Multiple Sclerosis*. New York: Franklin Watts, 2000.
Burnett, Betty, and Rob Gevertz. *Coping with Multiple Sclerosis*. New York: Rosen, 2001.

# ■ MUSCULAR DYSTROPHY

*See*: Genetic Disorders

# ■ OBESITY

A **chronic** disorder in which body weight exceeds the norm by 30 percent or more. The Centers for Disease Control and Prevention define *overweight* as having a **body mass index (BMI)** of 25 to 29.9 and *obese* as having a BMI of 30 or more.

Children are overweight if the BMI is greater than or equal to the 95 percentile for their age. BMI is a formula for measuring ideal weight. It uses your height to adjust for your weight as it compares you to other individuals and populations. For example, two teens might each weigh 150 pounds, but one might be five feet tall

## DID YOU KNOW?

# How Overweight and Obesity Are Diagnosed

The most common way to find out whether you're overweight or obese is to figure out your body mass index (BMI). BMI is an estimate of body fat and a good gauge of your risk for diseases that occur with more body fat. The higher your BMI, the higher your risk of disease.

# Body Mass Index for Adults

| Height | 21 | 22 | 23 | 24 | 25 | 26 | 27 | 28 | 29 | 30 | 31 |
|---|---|---|---|---|---|---|---|---|---|---|---|
| 4'10" | 100 | 105 | 110 | 115 | 119 | 124 | 129 | 134 | 138 | 143 | 148 |
| 5'0" | 107 | 112 | 118 | 123 | 128 | 133 | 138 | 143 | 148 | 153 | 158 |
| 5'1" | 111 | 116 | 122 | 127 | 132 | 137 | 143 | 148 | 153 | 158 | 164 |
| 5'3" | 118 | 124 | 130 | 135 | 141 | 146 | 152 | 158 | 163 | 169 | 175 |
| 5'5" | 126 | 132 | 138 | 144 | 150 | 156 | 162 | 168 | 174 | 180 | 186 |
| 5'7" | 134 | 140 | 146 | 153 | 159 | 166 | 172 | 178 | 185 | 191 | 198 |
| 5'9" | 142 | 149 | 155 | 162 | 169 | 176 | 182 | 189 | 196 | 203 | 209 |
| 6'0" | 150 | 157 | 165 | 172 | 179 | 186 | 193 | 200 | 208 | 215 | 222 |
| 6'1" | 159 | 166 | 174 | 182 | 189 | 197 | 204 | 212 | 219 | 227 | 235 |
| 6'3" | 168 | 176 | 184 | 192 | 200 | 208 | 216 | 224 | 232 | 240 | 248 |

You or your health-care provider can use this table or the National Heart, Lung, and Blood Institute's online BMI calculator to figure out your BMI. First, find your height on the far left column. Next, move across the row to find your weight. Once you've found your weight, move to the very top of that column. This number is your BMI.

Source: National Heart, Lung, and Blood Institute.

and the other six feet tall. Weight alone is a poor indicator of obesity.

You can calculate your BMI with a standard table. The index does have some limits though: It may overestimate the body fat of athletes or others who have a very muscular build or underestimate the body fat in older people or people who have lost muscle.

---

**DID YOU KNOW?**

# What Does Body Mass Index Mean?

## BMI

| | |
|---|---|
| 18.5–24.9 | Normal weight |
| 25.0–29.9 | Overweight |
| 30.0–39.9 | Obese |
| 40.0 and above | Extreme obesity |

BMI can be used for most men and women.

Source: National Heart, Lung, and Blood Institute.

---

### Body Mass Index for Children and Teens

Overweight is defined differently for children and teens than it is for adults. Because children are still growing, and boys and girls mature at different rates, BMIs for children and teens compare their heights and weights against growth charts that take age and sex into account. This is called BMI-for-age percentile. A child's or teen's BMI-for-age percentile shows how his or her BMI compares with other boys and girls of the same age.

What the BMI does not take into account is the distribution of body fat. Fat concentrated in the abdomen is much more dangerous than fat located under the skin. It also does not take into account that extra weight may be muscle mass and not fat.

Every day, a person expends energy through their resting **metabolism** plus the thermal effects of meals and physical activity. Obesity results when calorie intake consistently exceeds metabolic demands. Although the causes of this imbalance are not completely understood, they are thought to be both physiologic-genetic and environmental.

### CAUSES

An interaction of **genetics** and environmental factors is the most common cause of obesity. Studies show that **genes** can regulate food intake, alter energy expending, and control fat distribution in humans and other animals.

Many other factors can influence obesity. Psychological factors such as low self-esteem, mood disorders, **depression,** or binge-eating disorder can have an influence. Hormones also make a difference, and studies are currently under way to discern the role and method of the operation of hormones involved in appetite. Abnormal absorption of nutrients may also lead to obesity. Chronic tiredness can be a factor in obesity, because many people eat when they are tired, but not actually hungry, to maintain their energy levels and restore concentration. Some researchers believe that the body attempts to maintain the metabolic rate around a specific set point that may be controlled by the nervous system. Some people may have a higher than normal set point for body weight and for total amount of fat tissue in the body. Growth hormones and hormonal regulators such as **insulin** also are factors, as is a **sedentary** lifestyle or inactivity. Societal factors that favor inexpensive fast food high in fat and calories can also lead to obesity.

### PREVALENCE

One-third of American adults over age 20 are obese, and 60 percent are overweight. The number of seriously overweight children has tripled. Research shows that 51 percent of people in the United States do not get any regular physical exercise.

Obesity is associated with an increased prevalence of socioeconomic hardship due to a higher rate of disability, early retirement, and

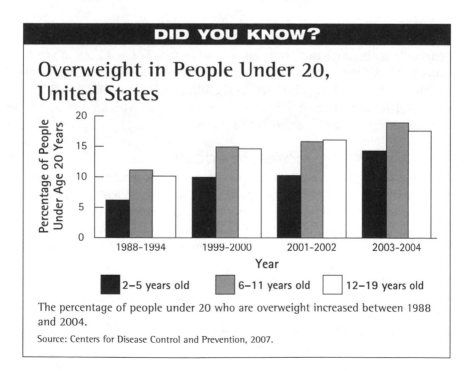

**DID YOU KNOW?**

## Overweight in People Under 20, United States

The percentage of people under 20 who are overweight increased between 1988 and 2004.

Source: Centers for Disease Control and Prevention, 2007.

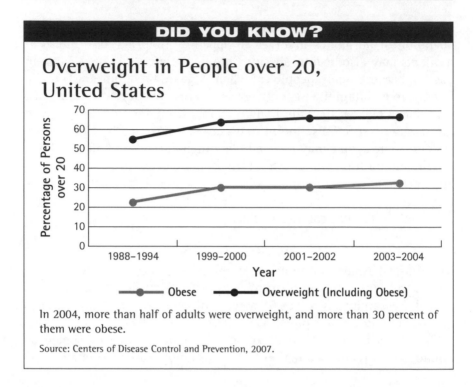

**DID YOU KNOW?**

## Overweight in People over 20, United States

In 2004, more than half of adults were overweight, and more than 30 percent of them were obese.

Source: Centers of Disease Control and Prevention, 2007.

widespread discrimination. An inverse relationship between socio-economic status and the prevalence of obesity has been documented, especially in women. Obesity in parents increases the probability of obesity in their children. Cultural and ethnic factors are also related to obesity. The incidence of obesity is high in female African-American, Native-American, and Latino populations.

## COMPLICATIONS

Problems arising from obesity include heart attack, stroke, **prediabetes**, diabetes, many types of cancer, Alzheimer's disease, macular degeneration, arthritis, osteoporosis, psoriasis, acne, depression, and attention deficit disorders. One estimate puts the health-care costs associated with obesity at $99 billion and 300,000 premature deaths each year.

### Prediabetes

Forty percent of people in the United States between the ages of 40 and 70 are prediabetic, and the prevalence of diabetes has tripled over the past two decades. Today, most patients in coronary care units are prediabetic or diabetic. Accumulation of fat in the abdomen leads to **insulin resistance,** the condition in which the body produces enough insulin for its needs, but the cells cannot use the insulin properly.

### Weight and Type 2 Diabetes Mellitus

Eighty percent of the people who develop Type 2 diabetes mellitus as adults are overweight. They have too much insulin in the blood, and the insulin does not work properly on body cells. As little as a 10 percent reduction in weight can reduce or eliminate abnormal blood sugar by normalizing the action of insulin.

### Cardiovascular Disease

Obesity increases the risk of **cardiovascular disease,** including hypertension, stroke, left ventricular hypertrophy, arrhythmias, congestive heart failure, myocardial infarction, angina pectoris, and peripheral vascular disease in both men and women. Mortality due to cardiovascular disease is 50 percent higher in obese people than in non-obese people; people with severe obesity have a 90 percent higher rate of mortality. In overweight people with hypertension, blood pressure will often return to normal with moderate weight loss.

### WEIGHT BIAS

One of the negative consequences of obesity in the United States is bias. In addition to bias in the media, cultural values connected to thinness are important in society. Self-control, hard work, and the delay of gratification are traditional American values; a thin body may be thought to symbolize hard work, ambition, desire, and control over eating impulses. The reverse side of this image is that overweight people are indulgent, lazy, and lacking control.

Although genetics and biology make it very hard for many to control their weight, the media and other societal avenues consistently send messages that the ideal human body is achievable if only you work hard enough and adopt the diet mentality.

Peer bullying and teasing research shows that 30 percent of overweight young girls and 24 percent of overweight young boys are teased at school. The chances of being teased increase with body weight, with 60 percent of those with the highest obesity reporting victimization by their schoolmates. The teasing and bullying from weight bias then make the obese children vulnerable to depression, **anxiety,** low self-esteem, poor body image, and suicidal thoughts and acts.

Weight bias can lead to unhealthy weight control and binge eating in those who are teased. Weight bias in women, research shows, can lead to overeating to cope with social stigma about weight. Another effect of weight bias is the avoidance of physical activity in settings where obese individuals are frequently victimized.

## TREATMENT

People spend more than $33 billion annually on weight-reduction products and services in the United States. Weight reduction and maintenance of optimal weight are treatment goals, which include a reduced-calorie diet, behavior modification, aerobic exercise, and social support.

Eating regularly throughout the day and keeping up with caloric needs rather than building a deficit and then overeating during the evenings is recommended. Studies show that eating breakfast with about 20 percent of the calories needed for the day is important to controlling weight. Typically, if breakfast is skipped, it starts a pattern of becoming preoccupied with thoughts of food later in the day and a loss of ability to sense when we are comfortably full. Ultimately, more calories are consumed by eating only in the evening than would have been consumed with planned, nutritious meals throughout the day.

A slow, steady loss of weight is preferred to crash or fad diet losses of more than 2.2 pounds per week. Drastic diets may produce rapid weight loss in the first weeks due to water loss, but the rate slows, and loss of much-needed muscle tissue will occur. During weight loss it is important to allow for slow changes in body composition and preservation of muscle mass by combining a well-balanced diet with exercise. Side effects can include later weight gain if muscle tissue is lost and no longer available to burn calories. Gall bladder disease is common in those who have rapidly lost and regained weight repeatedly.

In extreme instances where health is concerned, some patients pursue surgical weight loss, or bariatric surgery. This comes with risks and is done only after every other option is exhausted and significant weight reduction is necessary for one's survival.

*See also:* Anxiety and Mood Disorders; Chronic Disease; Diabetes Mellitus (DM); Genetic Disorders; Heart Disease

### FURTHER READING

Levy, Lance. *Understanding Obesity: The Five Medical Causes*. Buffalo, N.Y.: Firefly, 2000.

Normandi, Carol Emery, and Laurelee Roark. *It's Not about Food*. New York: Grosset/Putnam, 1998.

# ■ OSTEOPOROSIS

*See*: Obesity

# ■ PARKINSON'S DISEASE

A **chronic,** slowly progressive degeneration of the part of the brain and spinal cord that controls movement. Parkinson's is characterized by muscle rigidity and involuntary tremors. Eventually, performing daily activities causes fatigue and muscle cramp in the legs, neck, and trunk. Other symptoms are drooling, a masklike facial expression, loss of posture control when walking, and walking bent forward.

**Neurotransmitters** are substances that carry signals from one nerve cell to another. In Parkinson's, the damaged nerve cells do not produce the neurotransmitter **dopamine,** which releases a chemical that helps control muscle activity.

## CAUSE

Scientists now know that two **mutations,** or changes, in the **gene** for a protein cause the disease. Researchers continue to study how the gene mutations interact with other genes and with possible environmental factors. What causes the genes to mutate around age 60 isn't usually known. Because the disease selects only specific systems of nerve cells, scientists have ruled out poor circulation, **arteriosclerosis, infection,** and **inflammation** as causes. Some cases of Parkinson's are caused by exposure to toxins, such as manganese dust and carbon monoxide; another known cause is traumatic brain injury, such as that suffered by boxers.

## PREVALENCE

One of the most common crippling diseases in the United States, Parkinson's occurs in one of every 500 people over age 50. It affects males more often than it does females and usually occurs in middle age or later. The average age of onset is 60, but the early stages are gradual and include a slight sense of weakness with trembling in the hands and arms. It is difficult to date precisely when these symptoms begin. Over many years, the symptoms increase gradually and little change may be noticed from one year to another.

### TREATMENT

Drugs that target the area between nerve cells and manage the symptoms caused by a lack of dopamine are the mainstay of treatment for Parkinson's disease. The first group is called anticholinergic drugs. These are helpful in early stages and with minor symptoms such as tremor. Another group is dopaminergic drugs that give the patient a precursor to dopamine, which is then converted to dopamine inside the body. The patient may need to take a break from it, which then causes symptoms to return. Because the disease was progressing even as drugs were controlling the symptoms, a patient may experience even worse symptoms than before. A newer group of medications, the catechol O-methyltransferase (COMT) inhibitors, allow more of the dopaminergic drugs to get into the brain where they are needed.

In addition to medication, **physical therapy,** a healthful diet, and exercise can help people stay mobile and independent. You may have heard of other experimental approaches such as surgery or a device implanted in the brain to correct the signaling. None of these is standard treatment, but all of them are being seriously studied.

*See also:* Genetic Disorders

**FURTHER READING**
Duvoisin, Roger C., and Jacob Sage. *Parkinson's Disease.* 5th ed. Philadelphia: Lippincott Williams & Wilkins, 2001.

## ■ POST-TRAUMATIC STRESS DISORDER (PTSD)

*See*: Anxiety and Mood Disorders

## ■ RHEUMATOID ARTHRITIS

*See*: Arthritis

## ■ SCOLIOSIS

A disorder in which there is an S-shaped curve of the spine from the back view. The normal spine should be straight from the back view.

Scoliosis affects 2 percent of the population. Signs and symptoms are uneven shoulders, one shoulder blade more prominent than the other, uneven waist, one hip higher than the other, and leaning to one side. If the scoliosis gets worse, the spine will also rotate or twist. Most scoliosis begins during a growth spurt in adolescence. Because the spine is connected to the rib cage, rotation of the spine can cause a corresponding rotation of the rib cage; this rotation (curving) can be seen in the rib humps that develop in some scoliosis patients. The more the rib cage is rotated, the more it compresses the organs within it. So, some people develop heart problems or decreased lung capacity, lessening their ability to take deep breaths.

However, most scoliosis patients have only a mild degree of curvature and may not even need treatment. Suggested scoliosis treatments are dependent upon the combination of lateral curvature and rotation that a particular curve displays.

## PREVALENCE

Many people have such a minimal degree of curvature that its presence can go undetected. There are 25 scoliosis cases per 1,000 people. Females are much more likely to develop scoliosis than males. There is a higher incidence in families who have members with scoliosis, but no genetic link has been identified.

## COPING AND TREATMENT

If the curve is less than 20 degrees, as in the majority of scoliosis cases, no treatment is needed. Usually the health-care provider will do periodic exams and X-rays to make sure it does not worsen significantly. Many factors go into determining treatment. One option is wearing a brace. Usually used if the curve is 25–40 degrees, the brace will not cure scoliosis or reverse the curve, but it works to prevent progression and the need for surgery 90 percent of the time. One of the hardest parts of this treatment is having to wear the brace all day and night. However, it is key to this treatment working. Usually, the brace can be taken off to participate in activities or sports without restriction. A brace will not help after the spine has stopped growing—usually age 15–16 for girls and 17–18 for boys. There are two types of braces:

- Underarm or low-profile brace—this close-fitting plastic brace is almost invisible under clothes.
- Milwaukee brace—full body brace with a neck ring; it's much larger and rarely used today.

# Q & A

**Question: How effective is bracing in treating scoliosis?**

**Answer:** Braces do not cure scoliosis, but they slow and sometimes stop scoliosis curves from progressing to higher degrees of curvature. In patients with curves of 20–40 degrees, studies have shown braces to be effective if worn for the prescribed number of hours. Some people have curves that cannot be controlled by bracing and some need surgery right away.

Surgery is complicated and involves fusing the vertebrae together to prevent the spine from curving any further. It is usually done only when the curve is greater than 40–50 degrees.

**FURTHER READING**

Lyons, Brooke, Oheneba Boachie-Adjei, John Podzius, and Carla Podzius. *Scoliosis: Ascending the Curve.* New York: Evans, 1999.

## ■ SEXUALLY TRANSMITTED DISEASES (STDS)

Diseases that are spread through sexual activity. Both **bacteria** and **viruses** cause STDs. Bacterial STDs can be treated with **antibiotics,** and there are **vaccines** to prevent some viral STDs. Most are curable with early detection and treatment, but some cause few distinctive symptoms. Some cannot be cured and lead to life-threatening complications.

The surest way to avoid STDs is to abstain from sexual contact or to be in a long-term mutually monogamous relationship with a partner who has been tested and shown to be uninfected. In some STDs, the use of latex condoms reduces the risk of transmission.

HIV, the virus that causes AIDS, is an STD, and it can increase the risk of contracting other STDs as well. People with STDs are two to five times more likely than those without STDs to be infected if exposed to HIV. Also, people infected with HIV who also have another STD are more likely to transmit HIV through sexual contact than those with HIV who do not have another STD. In both cases, having one disease may compromise one's **immune system,** increasing one's susceptibility to getting another disease.

## DID YOU KNOW?

# Occurrence and Prevalence of the Most Common STDs

In the United States alone, as of 2004, an estimated 19 million new cases of STDs were reported each year.

| STD | Incidence* | Prevalence** |
|---|---|---|
| Chlamydia | 2,800,000 | *** |
| Gonorrhea | 700,000 | *** |
| Syphilis | 32,000 (reported) | *** |
| Herpes (HSV) | 1,000,000 | 45,000,000 |
| Hepatitis B (HBV) | 60,000 | 1,250,000 |
| Genital Warts / Human Papillomavirus (HPV) | 6,200,000 | 20,000,000 |
| Trichomoniasis | 7,400,000 | *** |

* Estimated number of new cases each year
** Estimated number of people currently infected
*** No recent surveys on national prevalence for gonorrhea, syphilis, chlamydia, or trichomoniasis have been conducted.

STDs affect men and women of all backgrounds and economic levels. However, STDs disproportionately affect women and infants of infected women.

Source: Centers for Disease Control and Prevention, 2004.

Bacteria cause STDs such as **chlamydia**, syphilis, and gonorrhea. Hepatitis B, hepatitis C, genital herpes, and genital HPV are common STDs caused by viruses.

### CHLAMYDIA

Chlamydia is an STD caused by a bacterium that can damage a woman's reproductive organs. Known as the "silent disease," chlamydia causes no symptoms in most women and half of the men infected. Women who do have symptoms experience abnormal vaginal discharge or a burning sensation when urinating. Later, as the infection spreads farther into the reproductive system, women might experience lower abdominal pain, lower back pain, nausea, and fever. Men with symptoms experience penile discharge or burning upon urination.

Chlamydia can affect any sexually active person. Treatment includes antibiotics for the infected person and any sex partners of that person. Additionally, persons with chlamydia should abstain from sexual intercourse until treatment is completed to avoid spreading the disease.

## SYPHILIS

An STD caused by a bacterium, the number of syphilis cases increased almost 12 percent in 2005. The bacteria are spread from one person to another through direct contact with syphilis sores, which mainly occur on the external genitals, vagina, anus, or in the rectum. There are three stages of syphilis infection, and the disease can be transmitted before any symptoms appear.

Primary stage: About 21 days after infection, one or more sores (chancres) appear at the site of infection. Lasting three to six weeks, the chancre(s) heal without treatment; without treatment, though, infection goes to the next stage.

Secondary stage: Signs of the second stage are rashes and mucous membrane lesions. Additional symptoms that can appear are fever, swollen lymph glands, sore throat, hair loss, headaches, weight loss, fatigue, and muscle aches. Again, the symptoms of syphilis will disappear without treatment; without treatment, syphilis enters the next stage.

Latent and late stages: In the latent, or hidden, stage, the infection can remain in the body for years with no apparent symptoms. About 15 percent of people with untreated syphilis develop symptoms in the late stage, which can occur as much as 20 years after the initial infection. Damage to vital internal organs happens in the late stage as do symptoms of difficulty with movement, paralysis, numbness, gradual blindness, and **dementia**. The chancres of syphilis can break and make it easier for transmission of HIV infection.

Syphilis is easily cured in its early stages with penicillin or other antibiotics if the patient is allergic to penicillin. People with syphilis sores must abstain from sexual contact until the sores are completely healed. It is important for people with behaviors that put them at risk for acquiring STDs be screened regularly for syphilis.

## GONORRHEA

Another STD caused by a bacterium is gonorrhea, which easily multiplies in women's reproductive tracts including the cervix, uterus, and fallopian tubes (egg canals), and in the urethras of women and men. It also grows in the mouth, throat, eyes, and anus. Gonorrhea is spread through contact with the vagina, penis, mouth, or anus.

The CDC estimates that 700,000 people each year contract gonorrhea. People at highest risk are teens, young adults, and African Americans, though any sexually active person can be infected.

Complications of the disease for women are pelvic inflammatory disease (PID), which can result in **chronic** pelvic pain, infertility, and a risk of ectopic pregnancy, in which a fertilized egg grows outside the uterus. In men, infertility is also a complication. In both genders, a life-threatening infection of the blood or **joints** can happen, and people with gonorrhea can more easily get and transmit HIV. Gonorrhea is cured with antibiotics, but drug-resistant strains are increasing worldwide, making treatment more challenging.

## HEPATITIS B

Caused by a virus that attacks the liver, hepatitis B can cause **cirrhosis** of the liver, liver cancer, liver failure, and death. The virus is transmitted through the blood of an infected person during sex without condom use, sharing of drugs or needles, or from an infected mother to her baby during birth. Thirty percent of people with hepatitis B have no symptoms; symptoms are **jaundice** (yellowish color), fatigue, abdominal pain, loss of appetite, nausea, vomiting, and joint pain. The best protection is the hepatitis B vaccine. Using latex condoms might reduce transmission. Never using or sharing drugs and needles, never sharing personal care items, and not getting tattoos or body piercings are ways to prevent getting hepatitis B.

## HEPATITIS C

Transmitted through blood and body fluids or contracted during tattooing or by the sharing of needles by drug users, hepatitis C accounts for about 20 percent of all viral hepatitis cases. The 50 to 80 percent of people infected with hepatitis C that have a chronic condition are **infectious**. Liver cancer is a possible complication. Although there is no vaccine against hepatitis C, there are several drugs that effectively treat it. In early stages of the disease, resting and eating small, high-calorie, high-protein meals promote recovery.

## GENITAL HERPES

The herpes simplex viruses type 1 (HSV-1) or type 2 (HSV-2) cause genital herpes, an STD that has no or few symptoms. When the symptoms do appear, they are blisters on or around the genitals or rectum. The blisters break and then heal within two to four weeks. HSV-1 and

HSV-2 can be released from the sores, but they are released between outbreaks from skin that does not have sores. HSV-1 and HSV-2 can be released between outbreaks when the person is unaware of a sore and he or she can spread the virus through sexual contact. HSV-2 infection is transmitted only through sexual contact with someone who has the virus. People diagnosed with a first episode of genital herpes will typically have four or five outbreaks in a year. Over time, outbreaks will decrease in frequency. One out of five adolescents and adults, or 45 million people in the United States, have had genital HSV infection. These are new antiviral medications used to treat outbreaks, reduce symptoms, and genital sores. Some patients take these medications daily to avoid affecting their partner.

## GENITAL HPV INFECTION

The most common sexually transmitted infection is genital human papillomavirus (HPV), which infects the skin and mucous membranes of the genital areas of men and women. Transmitted through genital contact, HPV does not cause symptoms and health problems, so most people are unaware that they are infected and pass the virus to a partner. Low-risk types cause warts and high-risk types cause cancer. In both low- and high-risk types, the immune system clears the HPV infection within two years.

In the United States, 6.2 million people are newly infected with HPV each year, and approximately 50 percent of sexually active people are infected with HPV at some time. A vaccine can protect females from the types of HPV that cause most cervical cancers and genital warts, which appear as small bumps in the genital area. **Vaccination** is recommended for 11- and 12-year-old girls and women 13 through 26 who have not completed the vaccine series. Condoms may lower the risk of developing diseases related to HPV, but are not fully protective, so avoiding sexual activity is the only sure prevention.

*See also:* AIDS (Acquired Immunodeficiency Syndrome); Centers for Disease Control and Prevention (CDC); Hepatitis; Immunization; Infections, Bacterial and Viral; Skin Disorders

### FURTHER READING

Haerens, Margaret, ed. *Sexually Transmitted Diseases*. Detroit: Greenhaven, 2007.
Woods, Samuel G. *Everything You Need to Know about STDs*. New York: Rosen, 2003.

# ■ SICKLE-CELL DISEASE
*See*: Genetic Disorders

# ■ SKIN DISORDERS
Diseases of the body's largest organ system, the skin. The skin performs many important functions, including protecting the structures beneath it, regulating temperature and blood pressure, perceiving the environment, synthesizing vitamin D, and excreting sweat. The severity of skin disorders can range from minor irritations to fatality. Causes of skin disorders are heredity, **viruses,** environment, and hormones.

## ACNE
Acne is defined as plugged pores (blackheads and whiteheads), pimples, and deep lumps that occur on the upper body. Almost 100 percent of people between 12 and 17 have had at least a whitehead, blackhead, or pimple. In most cases, acne lasts for five to 10 years and goes away on its own when people are in their 20s. There are people who suffer from acne in later adult years, though. Although it is not a life-threatening condition, it can be upsetting, and even less severe cases can leave scars.

Although many people believe that eating foods such as chocolate, french fries, and pizza can cause acne, there is no scientific evidence supporting a connection of diet to acne.

# Fact Or Fiction?

### Acne is caused by not keeping skin clean enough.

**The Facts:** Acne is not caused by dirty or oily skin. Washing the skin too vigorously and frequently can actually irritate the skin and make acne worse. Dermatologists recommend gently washing the face twice daily with mild soap, patting the skin dry, and using a topical treatment for acne. Neither blackheads nor whiteheads should be squeezed open, because if tissues are injured, **bacteria** can cause infections at the site.

## WARTS
The human papillomavirus (HPV) causes warts, which are growths on the top layer of skin. If the skin has been damaged in some way—by people biting their nails, for instance—warts can infect more easily.

Common warts grow on the fingers, around nails and on the backs of hands. They usually occur where skin is broken. Plantar warts grow on the soles of the feet and are flat due to body weight pushing them back into the skin. Flat warts are smaller and smoother than other warts but grow in large numbers (20–100 at a time.)

Over-the-counter treatments are available for warts, and dermatologists have a variety of treatments, including new laser and **immunotherapy** treatments.

## COLD SORES

Cold sores, or fever blisters, are causes by herpes simplex virus (HSV type 1). Most often occurring on the face, cold sores are small, fluid-filled blisters. The virus usually spreads among family members or friends and can be transmitted by kissing, sharing eating utensils, or by sharing towels.

Herpes simplex virus type 2 (HSV type 2), usually transmitted through sexual intercourse, results in sores on the buttocks, penis, vagina, or cervix. Up to 20 percent of all sexually active adults in the United States, or between 5 million and 20 million people, are affected by HSV-2.

### Treatment and Prevention

Herpes infections are treated with antiviral medications. In addition to treating outbreaks, the medications can suppress herpes outbreaks from recurring. When there is tingling, burning, itching, or tenderness of a body area with a herpes infection, that area should be kept away from other people to prevent contagion. People with mouth herpes should avoid kissing and sharing drinking cups and lip balms. People with genital herpes should avoid sexual relations during periods of symptoms and always use condoms. It is estimated that 80 percent of all genital herpes is transmitted when there are no lesions or symptoms.

## INHERITED SKIN DISEASES

Psoriasis and keratosis pilaris (dry skin) are skin disorders that are inherited. The **genes** that cause psoriasis determine reactions of the **immune system**. A trigger such as stress, sunburn, injury to the skin, and some medications can cause psoriasis. Symptoms of psoriasis are patches of raised, reddish skin covered by white scales that cause discomfort. The skin may itch and may crack and bleed. There is no cure for this **chronic** condition.

Keratosis pilaris occurs more often as people age, in winter, and in low-humidity climates. The skin becomes dry from lack of water, not oil, so taking in water orally to replace water in the skin is the focus of treatment.

## SKIN CANCER

Skin cancer is usually detectable in early stages because the tumor of replicated cells with damaged DNA develops on the outer layer of the skin and can be seen. Exposure to the Sun's UV rays, which damage DNA in the skin, is the leading cause of cancer, and many cases of cancer could be prevented with protection from the Sun. Usually the body can repair the Sun damage before genes mutate and cancer develops, but with cumulative sun exposure, cancer develops.

Basal cell skin cancer is the most common form of skin cancer. Ninety percent of tumors occur on Sun-exposed areas of the body. Found on the top layer of skin, this cancer can be successfully removed if found early enough.

Squamous cell skin cancer forms a little deeper, in the squamous cells of the skin, usually on the face, lips, and nose. Still, if caught early enough, it can be removed successfully.

Melanoma is the most dangerous and deadly form of skin cancer. Formed in the deeper melanocyte, or melanin, skin cells, it can more easily get to and travel through the lymph system to other areas of the body before becoming a noticeable problem. Interestingly, this skin cancer can often be found on body areas with less Sun exposure, such as the abdomen or back, even though the entire body's exposure to Sun is a risk factor. Tanning beds, which use UV (B or A) rays, are a risk particularly in this type of skin cancer because the rays go deeper into the melanin cells to tan the skin.

Melanoma treatment can be quite complex. If caught early, surgical removal may be all that is necessary, but due to the deeper cells, scars may be more severe. Additionally, if the cancer has spread, interferon or other drug treatments may be prescribed.

Anyone of any color can develop skin cancer, but those with the most risk are those with fair skin, light-colored eyes, blond or red hair, a tendency to burn or freckle, and a history of Sun exposure. Anyone with a family history of skin cancer is also at risk.

Most people do not protect their skin from the Sun's harmful rays, and if current trends continue, one in five people in the United States will develop skin cancer. Sun protection includes staying out of the Sun between 10 A.M. and 4 P.M. when the Sun's rays are strongest, wearing sunscreen, and wearing protective clothing.

*See also:* Cancer; Centers for Disease Control and Prevention (CDC); Chronic Disease; Infections, Bacterial and Viral; Sexually Transmitted Diseases (STDs)

**FURTHER READING**

Kenet, Barney, and Patricia Lawler. *Saving Your Skin: Prevention, Early Detection, and Treatment of Melanoma and Other Skin Cancers, 2nd Edition.* New York City: Four Walls Eight Windows, 1998.

McClay, Edward, Mary-Eileen McClay, and Jodie Smith. *100 Questions & Answers About Melanoma & Other Skin Cancers.* Boston: Jones and Bartlett Publishers, 2003.

Schofield, Jill, and William Robinson. *What You Really Need to Know About Moles and Melanoma.* Baltimore: John Hopkins Press, 2000.

Sutton, Amy, ed. *Dermatological Disorders Sourcebook: Basic Consumer Health Information about Conditions and Disorders Affecting Skin, Hair, and Nails, 2nd Ed.* Detroit: Omnigraphics, 2005.

Turkington, Carol, and Jeffrey Dover. *Encyclopedia of Skin and Skin Disorders.* New York: Facts On File, 2002.

Turkington, Carol, and Jeffrey Dover. *Skin Deep: An A-Z of Skin Disorders, Treatment, and Health.* New York: Facts On File, 1998.

# ■ STREP INFECTIONS

Diseases caused by the bacterium *Streptococcus pyogenes,* or Group A beta-hemolytic streptococcus. Some of the diseases are mild, such as strep throat (pharyngitis), but some Group A streptococci have caused deadly epidemics.

Found only in humans, the **bacteria** usually reside in the nose and throat, and occasionally on the skin. Transmitted through person-to-person contact, they spread though the air as fluid droplets leave the nose or throat during sneezing or speaking or by sharing eating utensils or drinking glasses. School-age children have the highest incidence of infection, and infection in the winter months is most common.

## STREP THROAT

Strep throat, a painful **inflammation** of the throat, is one of the most costly **infectious** diseases in the world. Most often, sore throats are caused by **viruses.** In 15 percent of sore throats, a strain of Group A streptococcus causes strep throat. Symptoms of strep are fever above 101°F (38.3°C), chills, aches, lack of appetite, nausea, and vomiting. Tonsils may be swollen and red and may be dotted with white or yellow spots. Viral pharyngitis, or sore throat caused by a virus instead of the strep bacteria, has symptoms of a sore throat and mild fever. Most health-care providers will do a quick test in the office to help determine if the cause is strep.

The **incubation period,** the time between first exposure to the bacteria and the development of strep throat, is two to seven days. The fever then lasts three to five days, with the sore throat fading afterward. If the strep is untreated, the infected person is **contagious,** able to pass the bacteria on to others, from the first exposure to the disappearance of symptoms. If **antibiotics** are taken, the person is no longer contagious after starting the antibiotics.

Between 10 and 20 percent of children are estimated to be **carriers** of the bacteria but do not show outward signs of the disease. Generally, the bacteria are transmitted to close contacts only, but occasionally epidemics occur.

### IMPETIGO

Impetigo is a skin infection that can be caused by Group A streptococci. Most common in preschool and school-age children, impetigo has symptoms of small skin blisters on the face, mouth, and nose that yellow and crust as they heal. If scratching causes the blisters to burst, bacteria on the hands can spread the disease to other areas or other people. The bacteria can also spread by touching infected clothing and towels. About two days after starting antibiotics to treat the impetigo the infected person ceases to be contagious. The best way to prevent the disease is by frequent hand washing.

### SCARLET FEVER

No longer as common as it was throughout most of recorded history, scarlet fever today is rarely fatal. Children with scarlet fever develop symptoms of chills, aches, loss of appetite, nausea, and vomiting after or while they have sore throats. A rash starts as itchy small bumps appear and spread over the body. Then the bumps merge together; the tonsils and back of the throat may be covered with a whitish coating and may appear swollen and red; the tongue may have a whitish coating and turn red ("strawberry tongue") as its surface begins to peel. Treatment is bed rest and 10 days of antibiotics.

### TOXIC SHOCK SYNDROME (TSS)

**Toxic shock syndrome** is a serious infection that came to attention in the 1980s. There are two types of TSS. When tampons were first linked to the infection, the particular type of tampon thought to cause the infection was removed from stores. However, it was discovered that *staphylococcus aureus* bacteria is the cause of this type of TSS, and anyone who has any type of staph infection, such as pneumonia or a skin infection, can get TSS.

The second type of infection is streptococcal toxic shock syndrome, STSS, and this is caused by a streptococcus bacteria. The skin is the usual route of entry for this infection.

STSS is an example of an invasive disease, one in which the microbe has gotten past the body's outer defenses and gotten into the bloodstream and spread throughout the body. In STSS, the infection usually began at a cut, scrape, or bruise.

Severe pain and fever is the most common first symptom of STSS. In 10 percent of patients, a rash similar to scarlet fever may be present. As blood pressure drops rapidly, shock and organ failure can occur. In 80 percent of people with STSS, the soft tissue may be infected and may lead to a fatal deep tissue infection.

## RHEUMATIC FEVER

After a strep infection is gone, and the bacteria are killed, sometimes the worst effects of the strep bacteria appear. One example of this is rheumatic fever, which comes after sore throats caused by some strains of Group A streptococci. After half a century of decline in incidence, rheumatic fever resurged in the 1980s with three epidemics in the United States. Although the incidence of rheumatic fever has increased in recent decades, deaths are rare from the disease.

Most frequently striking children between five and 15, rheumatic fever has symptoms of fever and arthritis. Rheumatic fever can damage heart valves, causing them to open or close incorrectly, which allows blood to leak and the heart to pump harder. If the heart damage is permanent, the condition is called rheumatic heart disease. Occurring in about half of rheumatic fever patients, it occurs within three weeks of the start of symptoms. Rheumatic fever and rheumatic heart disease happen most often in developing countries. If rheumatic fever has severely damaged the heart valves, surgery may be required to replace them with animal or artificial valves.

Scientists are researching several strategies for developing an effective **vaccine** against Group A streptococcus. Because it would likely save 400,000 lives lost each year worldwide to rheumatic fever and rheumatic heart disease alone, there is great interest in such a vaccine.

*See also:* Heart Disease; Immunization; Infections, Bacterial and Viral; Treatment

### FURTHER READING

Smith, Tara. *Streptococcus (Group A).* Deadly Diseases and Epidemics. Philadelphia: Chelsea House, 2005.

# ■ STROKE

*See*: Heart Disease

# ■ STREPTOCOCCAL TOXIC SHOCK-LIKE SYNDROME

*See*: Infections, Bacterial and Viral

# ■ TREATMENT

A course of action to fight illness or disease that is specific to the symptoms and nature of the disease. Careful diagnosis is essential to successfully prescribing a plan of treatment. Different specialists might even approach the same disease differently.

Medical advances of the 20th century increased life expectancy for Americans from 47 years in 1900 to 77 years in 2000. Formerly untreatable diseases such as whooping cough and diphtheria, which took many lives, especially those of children, became preventable with vaccines. With technological improvements of the 20th century, doctors increased the effectiveness of their diagnoses and surgeries. Tuberculosis, which caused 20 deaths per 10,000 people in 1900, is today nearly nonexistent. Pneumonia and influenza caused about 20 deaths per 10,000 people; today, medicines to treat their symptoms make them much less of a threat—two deaths per 10,000 people. In the United States, life expectancy for females in 2005 is more than 80 years; life expectancy for males is about 75 years. Some scientists are predicting the extension of life expectancy will increase for an average life span of 100 years for those who stay active, eat a nutritious diet, and do not smoke or engage in risky behaviors.

## CLASSES OF DRUGS

Different kinds of drugs are used to fight different types of infections. Viral infections cannot be treated with **antibiotics,** for instance. This is why it is important for a health-care professional to diagnose an illness and prescribe medication. They know which medications will be effective against each type of disease.

### Antibiotics

Some of the most widely used medications today, antibiotics are classified by the action they exert in stopping **bacteria.** For example, beta-lactam antibiotics attach to cell receptors, preventing new bacterial cells from being made. Penicillin is one of the beta-lactams. Certain antibiotics target certain kinds of bacteria. For example, penicillin treats a bacteria called gram-positive cocci. Other antibiotics work in other ways and on other kinds of bacteria.

An increasing problem is overuse of antibiotics for nonbacterial infections such as sinus infections, 80 percent of which are caused by viruses. Then, when a true bacterium causes an infection, the antibiotic may not work effectively or at all.

## Vaccines
Vaccines have saved millions of lives and kept millions from the complications of diseases such as polio. Vaccines provide two types of immunization: passive and active. Passive immunization is a vaccine of antibodies against a specific antigen, or it can occur naturally due to the general set of antibodies most people would have. Active immunization is a vaccine made of a killed pathogen, which causes the body to make antibodies to the infection. If the body comes in contact with the bacterium again, the body will have antibodies ready to kill the bacterium.

## Cardiovascular Medications
Cardiovascular disease, or heart disease, is the number one cause of death in the United States, and medications to treat it have increased dramatically. Statins, a group of drugs, are now a mainstay in the treatment of high cholesterol, which factors in heart disease. Statins have been shown to reduce heart attacks and death from heart attacks.

Several groups of drugs to treat hypertension have been discovered, and each one treats a different part of the condition that is hypertension. Several drugs treat two things at once: Beta blockers have been shown to reduce the likelihood of a second heart attack regardless of blood pressure, so they are a standard drug for heart patients. But they can be used to treat the person's high blood pressure at the same time.

Newer drugs to prevent clots from forming where a previous clot has been have become standard treatment for at least one year after a heart attack. Aspirin is also standard treatment for prevention of first or subsequent heart attacks because of its anticlotting feature.

## Psychotropic drugs
Psychotropic drugs, medicines to treat mental illness, have greatly improved people's lives. Drugs for depression, bipolar disorder, and

schizophrenia may allow people to live productive lives. Before these therapies, some of these patients were outcasts and often locked away in facilities for years.

### Pain Medications

There are a wide range of medications for pain control. One of the oldest and simplest medications is aspirin. Newer drugs attempt to reduce pain and **inflammation** as aspirin does without some of its side effects, such as bleeding and heartburn. However, simple aspirin is still one of the most widely used pain medications in the world. On the other end of the spectrum, narcotics may be needed for severe pain such as that after surgery or cancer pain. Cancer patients used to suffer with pain until death, but now terminal cancer patients can usually live out their lives with much better pain control, as newer narcotics have been developed.

## CHEMOTHERAPY

**Chemotherapy** is the use of drugs to treat cancer. The drugs destroy cancer cells without permanently damaging the normal cells of the body. Cancer cells are unable to repair themselves after they are damaged. Chemotherapy destroys small tumors or shrinks larger tumors.

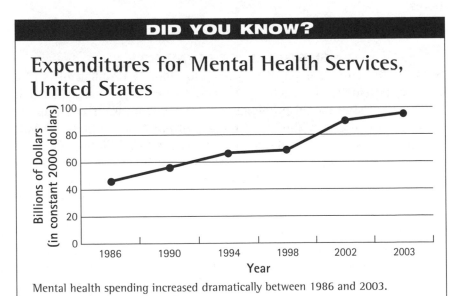

**DID YOU KNOW?**

## Expenditures for Mental Health Services, United States

Mental health spending increased dramatically between 1986 and 2003.

Source: Substance Abuse and Mental Health Services Administration; Chartbook on Trends in the Health of Americans, 2007.

If surgery is used to remove tumors, chemotherapy can be used afterward to destroy cancer cells that have spread to other parts of the body. Chemotherapy is used to cure cancer, prevent cancer from spreading, slow the cancer's growth, and relieve symptoms.

Some chemotherapy drugs kill cells by affecting the cell division process. Other drugs give the cancer cells a negative environment.

## Q & A

**Question: What are the side effects of chemotherapy?**

**Answer:** Each person responds differently to the drug treatments, but physical symptoms experienced by many people undergoing chemotherapy include hair loss, diarrhea, constipation, fatigue, anemia, infection, mouth and throat discomfort, and dryness of skin and nails. Your health-care provider can suggest ways to relieve any discomfort from side effects and can prescribe treatment for those side effects that could be a further health threat.

Emotional side effects could include depression and stress. These side effects can be treated through support groups and counseling, which can help you identify personal strategies for achieving realistic goals.

### SURGICAL TREATMENTS

Surgery, the cutting open of the body to repair a problem or cure a disease, is usually preceded by X-rays, two-dimensional scans that show hard tissue (bone) problems clearly, CT (**computerized tomography**) scans that can show 3-D images of parts of the body, or MRI (**magnetic resonance imaging**), which uses a combination of radio waves and a strong magnetic field to form an image of the inside of the body. MRI creates incredibly clear scans that do not expose the patient to radiation, and it has made a major impact on surgery.

### Microsurgery

**Microsurgery** involves operating while looking through glasses with magnifying lenses or microscopes; only a tiny hole, millimeters across, is needed for this surgery. It is used to repair arteries, veins, nerves, and muscles; one of its main uses is to reattach severed limbs.

### Laser Surgery

Laser light is a beam of concentrated, focused light. The laser material is a solid, liquid, or gas that is excited by electricity, and a beam of light is produced by light waves all moving the same direction. The lasers are precise and do not damage the nearby tissues. They work quickly, reducing the exposure to infection. They also can be used in microsurgery and cause less bleeding than traditional surgery.

In cancer, heat from lasers is used to cut off blood supply to tumors, and patients may be treated with chemicals that become poisonous to cells once they are exposed to laser light. Once the tumor cells soak up the chemicals, the laser is focused on the tumor, destroying it.

### Organ Transplants, Artificial Joints, and Valves

More than 21,000 organ transplants were done in the United States in 2007, and more than 12,000 of those were kidney transplants. Increasingly, as the population ages, surgeons are using artificial joints to replace hips, knees, and shoulders. When the valves of the heart that keep blood from flowing backward no longer function, a life-threatening condition develops. When this happens, an artificial plastic valve or a replacement valve from an animal or a human can be inserted.

## GENE THERAPY

Still in the experimental stage, gene therapy changes faulty genes or prevents them from being activated. This is used to treat, cure, or prevent diseases that result from faulty genes. Scientists know that single defective genes result in more than 3,000 diseases.

A defective gene will produce a defective protein or no protein at all. One treatment, called gene replacement therapy, gives the patient the missing or faulty protein that has been made by a genetically engineered bacteria to carry the properly functioning human gene.

## STEM CELL THERAPY

Stem cell therapy is based on the ability of cells of embryos (humans in the earliest stage of life after conception) to develop into every cell in the human body. Less than a week old, and smaller than a grain of rice, embryos are at the center of a controversy over whether destroying an embryo is valid even if it could cure diseases like cancer, heart disease, and Alzheimer's disease.

### Stem Cell Research

In October 2005, researchers changed embryonic stem cells into cancer-killing cells, which in the future may be effective in treating leukemia, a cancer of the blood.

In August 2001, scientists developed some insulin-making cells from embryonic stem cells. In the future, they hope that this may treat diabetes, a disease that interferes with the body's ability to make **insulin,** which controls the amount of glucose in the blood. Stem cells could be used to replace badly burned skin and treat brain disorders, such as Alzheimer's disease. Stem cells also have the potential to treat spinal cord injuries. Researchers with the American Heart Association theorize that adult stem cells could be used to treat heart disease, the major cause of death in the United States; studies show that brain function might be someday be restored to brain-damaged stroke victims. Adult stem cells are less able to change than embryonic stem cells, but they can repair moderate damage.

An adult stem cell is an undifferentiated cell—one whose purpose has not yet been defined by scientists. These cells are found in many organs and tissues in the human body, but there are very small amounts in the tissues of the brain, bone marrow, peripheral blood, blood vessels, skeletal muscle, skin, and liver. These cells stay in their static state for many years until disease or tissue injury activates them. Some scientists now use the term somatic stem cell instead of adult stem cell. Scientists are trying to find ways to grow adult stem cells so that they can use them to cure certain diseases such as Parkinson's disease and Type 1 diabetes.

Although ethical issues and potential rejection by the body's immune system limit the use of embryonic stem cells in medicine, scientists reported in fall 2007 that adult human skin cells may be a future source of stem cells with developmental capabilities and would have the same features as embryonic stem cells. Using four genes, scientists reprogrammed mouse cells to a state similar to that of embryonic stem cells. In the research, skin cells from mice were used to successfully correct a genetic defect for humanized sickle cells in mice. This points to a possible generation of stem cells from an individual patient to allow for producing cells affected by a patient's disease.

However, it remained unclear whether these "induced pluripotent stem cells" (iPS) can be produced directly from elderly patients with chronic diseases. In August 2008, scientists reported that iPS cells were produced from an 82-year-old woman with amyotrophic lateral sclerosis (ALS). Specific to this patient, the cells had the characteristics of embryonic stem cells and successfully differentiated into motor neurons, the cell type destroyed in ALS.

### Challenges

Stem cell researchers are faced not only with the ethical controversy of using embryonic stem cells, but with the possibility that both adult and embryonic stem cell therapies have the possibility of causing cancer. Another problem is the body's natural rejection of foreign substances; if adult stem cells could be made to change easily, a person's own stem cells could be used for treatment of a disease without that danger.

As society goes forward with the debate on using stem cells to treat disease, researchers look for ways to avoid the controversy in using stem cells from umbilical cord blood, which causes no harm to anyone and are not rejected by another person's body. Currently, there are umbilical cord blood banks storing lifesaving stem cells that may someday treat diseases.

## PSYCHOTHERAPY

Also called therapy or counseling, **psychotherapy** is a treatment based on talking and listening. Therapists are trained to treat emotional problems and help people figure out where a problem came from, help them fix the problem, and help them learn how to avoid future problems. Therapy is treatment for problems with parents and family, self-esteem, peers, and problems at school and work.

## PHYSICAL THERAPY

**Physical therapy** is the treatment of the muscles, bones, tendons, and ligaments of the body through reconditioning and strengthening the affected part. Often prescribed after orthopedic surgery, physical therapy treatment plans usually consist of a series of exercises and stretches. Sometimes the application of **ultrasound,** heat, ice, or massage may be done. The goal is to bring the person back to his or her normal level of functioning without further injury or pain.

## ALTERNATIVE MEDICINE

One type of alternative medicine involves natural treatments that rely on specific vitamins, herbs, and foods found in nature. Another is a system of beliefs and practices such as traditional Chinese medicine and **naturopathic** medicine that rely on natural treatments to help the body heal itself. Acupuncture, a form of traditional Chinese medicine, uses thin needles on specific points on the body to balance the body's energy. Advocates of this type of treatment use it to manage pain and nausea, increase circulation, and improve immune function. Some alternative treatments, such as Reiki or *qigong,* use energy fields to heal; others, such as yoga, prayer, music therapy, and meditation use the mind-body connection to heal. Massage therapy and chiropractic care involve stretching and manipulating various muscle and other tissue groups. Chiropractors adjust **joints,** usually the spine, so that they properly align. These therapies center on creating a sense of balance in the body and preventing illness.

Research shows that 36 percent of Americans use some form of alternative therapy. Before using alternative methods of treatment to relieve a problem, check with your family health-care provider or your parents or guardian to ensure the safety of the remedy. Substances in supplements or treatments can interact with drugs or foods that make them unsafe for you to use. Doctors or other adults can also help you research the alternative health-care provider's training and qualifications.

*See also:* AIDS (Acquired Immunodeficiency Syndrome); Cancer; Centers for Disease Control and Prevention (CDC); Chronic Disease; Heart Disease; Immunization; Infections, Bacterial and Viral; Strep Infections

**FURTHER READING**
Fullick, Ann. *Frontiers of Surgery.* Chicago: Heinemann, 2006.
Giddens, Sandra, and Owen Giddens. *Chemotherapy.* New York: Rosen, 2001.
Schacter, Bernice. *Biotechnology and Your Health: Pharmaceutical Applications.* Philadelphia: Chelsea House, 2006.

# ■ TUBERCULOSIS
*See*: Infections, Bacterial and Viral

# ■ TUMORS
*See*: Cancer; Treatment

# ■ VACCINES AND VACCINATIONS
*See*: Immunization

# HOTLINES AND HELP SITES

**Alateen**
URL: www.al-anon.alateen.org/alateen.html
Phone: (888) 4AL-ANON [8 a.m.–6 p.m. EST, M–F], (757) 563-1655
Fax: (757) 563-1655
Address: 1600 Corporate Landing Parkway, Virginia Beach, VA 23454-5617
Affiliation: Part of Al-Anon, an organization of relatives and friends of alcoholics
Mission: To help young people deal with problems of alcoholism in their families or among friends; members meet in small local groups to discuss their problems and provide mutual support
Program: Regular meetings of young people to discuss their problems and help one another face them

**Alcohol Treatment Referral Hotline**
Phone: (800) ALCOHOL [24 hours a day, 7 days a week]

**Alcoholics Anonymous**
URL: www.alcoholics-anonymous.org/index.cfm
Phone: (877) 934-2522, (212) 870-3400
Address: A.A. World Services, Inc., 475 Riverside Drive, 11th floor, New York, NY 10115
E-mail: publicinfo@aa.org
Mission: To stay sober and help other alcoholics achieve sobriety
Program: Worldwide fellowship of men and women from all walks of life who meet to attain and maintain sobriety

Alzheimer's Association
URL: www.alz.org/index.asp
Phone: (800) 272-3900 [24/7 helpline], (312) 335-8700
Address: Alzheimer's Association National Office, 225 North Michigan
  Avenue, 17th Floor, Chicago, IL 60601-7633
E-mail: info@alz.org
Mission: To eliminate Alzheimer's disease through the advance-
  ment of research, to provide and enhance care and support for all
  affected, and to reduce the risk of dementia through the promotion
  of brain health
Programs: Information, education, and support provided through the
  helpline, local chapters that offers core services to families and
  professionals, an online support community connecting people
  throughout the country, a 24-hour nationwide emergency response
  service for individuals with Alzheimer's disease or dementia, the
  nation's largest library devoted to Alzheimer's, an online suite
  of resources, a research grant program, a journal with the latest
  peer-reviewed research, programs to raise awareness of the disease,
  advocacy in Congress for Alzheimer's policy issues to increase federal funding for research of the disease

American Cancer Society
URL: www.cancer.org
Phone: (800) ACS-2345, (866) 228-4327
Mission: Dedicated to eliminating cancer as a major health problem by preventing cancer, saving lives, and diminishing suffering from cancer through research, education, advocacy, and
  service
Program: Community programs and services providing information
  on cancer prevention, early detection, treatment, survival, and
  quality of life, funding for research on cancer, and advocating for
  public policy concerning cancer

American Diabetes Association
URL: www.diabetes.org
Phone: (800) 232-3472
Mission: To prevent and cure diabetes and to improve the lives of all
  people affected by diabetes
Programs: Provides diabetes research, information, advocacy, and
  services to people with diabetes, their families, health professionals,
  and the public

**American Heart Association**
URL: www.americanheart.org
Phone: (800) AHA-USA1
Mission: To build healthier lives free of cardiovascular diseases and stroke
Programs: Support and provide advocacy for individuals, families, health-care professionals, and scientists in regards to cardiovascular diseases

**American Sickle-Cell Anemia Association**
URL: www.ascaa.org
Phone: (216) 229-8600
Address: 10300 Carnegie Avenue, Cleveland, OH 44106
E-mail: irabraqq@ascaa.org
Mission: To provide quality and comprehensive services to individuals and families at risk for sickle-cell disease
Programs: Provides diagnostic testing, evaluation, counseling, and supportive services; FAQs, support groups, multimedia

**Anorexia Nervosa and Related Eating Disorders, Inc.**
URL: www.anred.com
E-mail: Jarinor@rio.com
Mission: Provide information and resources on eating disorders
Programs: Information on many eating disorders; topics include definitions, warning signs, treatment and recovery, and ways to help a loved one

**Center for Infectious Disease Research and Policy, University of Minnesota**
URL: www.cidrap.umn.edu
Phone: (612) 626-6770
Address: University of Minnesota, Academic Health Center, 420 Delaware Street SE, MMC 263, Minneapolis, MN 55455
E-mail: Cidrap@umn.edu
Mission: Provides information and research
Programs: Content includes influenza, vaccines, avian flu, pandemic flu, food safety, SARS, and West Nile virus

**Center for Substance Abuse Treatment**
Phone: (800) 622-HELP
TDD: (800) 487-4889

Mission: To promote the quality and availability of community-based substance abuse treatment services for individuals and families who need them

Programs: Access to Recovery; Partners for Recovery; the Knowledge Application Program; the National Center on Substance Abuse and Child Welfare; National Alcohol and Drug Addiction Recovery Month; Substance Abuse Treatment Facility Locator; Medication Assisted Treatment; Recovery Community Services Program; CSAT's Addiction Technology Transfer Centers (ATTCs)

## Centers for Disease Control and Prevention
URL: www.cdc.gov
Phone: (800) CDC-INFO
Address: 1600 Clifton Road, Atlanta, GA 30333
E-mail: CDCinfo@cdc.gov
Mission: To strategize and plan for healthy people in every stage of life, preparedness for emerging health threats, and promote healthy people in a healthy world
Programs: Provide information about diseases and conditions, emergency preparedness and response, environmental health, life stages and populations, healthy living, injury, violence, safety, travelers' health, and workplace safety and health

## Centers for Disease Control and Prevention HIV/AIDS Hotline
URL: www.cdc.gov
Phone: (800) CDC-INFO
TTY: (888) 232-6348

## Childhelp USA
Phone: (800) 4-A-CHILD
Address: 15757 North 78th Street, Scottsdale, AZ 85260
Mission: Provide assistance for those dealing with child abuse

## Depression and Bipolar Support Alliance
URL: www.dbsalliance.org
Phone: (800) 826-3632, (800) 273-8255
Address: 730 North Franklin Street, Suite 501, Chicago, IL 60654-7225
Mission: To provide hope, help, support to improve the lives of people living with depression or bipolar disorder

Programs: Educational programs and events, e-newsletters, patient support groups, recovery education center, advocacy, reporting of research and clinical trials

Families for Depression Awareness
URL: www.familyaware.org
Phone: (781) 890-0220
Address: 395 Totten Pond Road, Suite 404, Waltham, MA 02451
E-mail: info@familyaware.org
Mission: To help families recognize and cope with depressive disorders to get people well and prevent suicide; help families recognize and manage various forms of depression and associated mood disorders; reduce stigma associated with depression; unite families and help them heal in coping with depression
Programs: Provide information and resources; distribute Family Profiles (interviews with people coping with depression); community outreach; awareness workshops; advocacy

Food and Nutrition Information Center
URL: www.nal.usda.gov/fnic
Address: National Agricultural Library, 10301 Baltimore Avenue, Room 105, Bestville, MD 20705
E-mail: fnic@nal.usda.gov
Mission: To be the leader in online global nutrition information
Programs: More than 2,000 links to current, reliable nutrition information; lending of resources; assistance in locating resources

Leukemia & Lymphoma Society
URL: www.leukemia-lymphoma.org
Phone: (800) 955-4572
Mission: To provide the latest research and treatment options in an education series and through a monthly society newsletter
Programs: Ongoing leukemia education series for patients, families, and health-care professionals

National Center for Learning Disabilities
URL: www.ncld.org
Phone: (212) 545-7510, (888) 575-7373
Address: 381 Park Avenue South, Suite 1401, New York, NY 10016

Mission: To ensure people with learning disabilities have every opportunity to succeed in school, work, and life

Programs: Information, resources and referral services; advocation for more effective policies; IDEA Watch published on Web site

## National Dissemination Center for Children with Disabilities (NICHCY)

URL: www.nichcy.org

Phone: (800) 695-0285

TTY: (202) 884-8200

Address: P.O. Box 1492, Washington, DC 20013

E-mail: nichcy@aed.org

Mission: To provide information about IDEA, No Child Left Behind, and effective educational practices concerning people with disabilities

Programs: Information about disabilities in children and youth, FAQs on Web site, and resource list for every state including parent training and information centers

## National Domestic Violence Hotline

URL: www.hduh.org

Phone: (800) 799-SAFE

TTY: (800) 787-3224

Program: A 24-hour call line to victims or anyone calling on their behalf that provides intervention, planning, safety information, and referrals.

## National Eating Disorders Association

URL: www.nationaleatingdisorders.org

Phone: (800) 931-2237, (206) 382-3587

Address: 603 Stewart Street, Suite 803, Seattle, WA 98101

E-mail: info@nationaleatingdisorders.org

Mission: Support individuals and families affected by eating disorders; serve as a catalyst for prevention, cures, and access to quality care

Programs: Campaign for prevention, improved access to quality treatment, and increased research funding to better understand and treat eating disorders and develop programs and tools to help everyone who seeks assistance

## National Hopeline Network

URL: www.hopeline.com

Phone: (800) SUICIDE

Mission: To aid those who have been contemplating suicide in finding help

## National Institute of Mental Health (NIMH)
URL: www.nimh.nih.gov
Phone: (301) 443-4513, (866) 615-6464
Address: Science Writing, Press and Dissemination Branch, 6001 Executive Boulevard, Room 8184, MSC 9663, Bethesda, MD 20892-9663
Mission: To reduce the burden of mental illness and behavioral disorders through research on the mind, brain, and behavior
Program: Supports the science of brain and behavior as a foundation for understanding mental disorders; defines genetic and environmental risk factors; develops tests and biomarkers for mental disorders; develops safe, effective, equitable treatments; supports clinical trials; and rapidly disseminates science information and services to mental health–care professionals

## National Institutes of Health: The Nation's Medical Research Agency
URL: www.nih.gov
Phone: (301) 496-4000
TTY: (301) 402-9612
Address: 9000 Rockville Pike, Bethesda, MD 20892
E-mail: NIHinfo@od.nih.gov
Mission: To help lead important medical discoveries that improve people's health and save lives; NIH scientists investigate ways to prevent disease and causes, treatments, and cures for common and rare diseases
Program: As part of the U.S. Department of Health and Human Services, NIH is the primary federal agency for conducting and supporting medical research; program areas include child and teen health, men's health, minority health, senior health, women's health, and wellness and lifestyle issues

## National Suicide Prevention Lifeline
URL: www.suicidepreventionlifeline.org
Phone: (800) 273-TALK
Program: Provides a 24-hour, toll free suicide prevention service available to those in suicidal crisis. The call is free and confidential.

**National Teen Dating Abuse**
URL: www.loveisrespect.org
Helpline: (866) 331-9474
TTY: (866) 331-8453
Program: Provides information and support to those dealing with teen
dating abuse.

**Organized Chaos**
URL: www.ocfoundation.org/organizedchaos/index.php
Phone: (617) 973-5801
Address: Obsessive-Compulsive Foundation, Inc., P.O. Box 961029,
Boston, MA 02196
Mission: To collaborate with Obsessive Compulsive Foundation, vari-
ous OCD experts, and contributing teens with OCD to help teens
and young adults with OCD through a webzine
Programs: Web site specifically for teens and young adults with
OCD

**The President's Council on Physical Fitness and Sports**
URL: www.fitness.gov
Phone: (202) 690-9000
Address: PCPFS Department W, 200 Independence Avenue SW, Room
738-H, Washington, DC 20201-0004
E-mail: hitness@HHS.gov
Mission: To provide information on health, physical activity, fitness,
and sports to achieve optimal physical fitness
Programs: Publications, challenge activities, interactive Web site, and
information on how to start physical activity programs

**Rape, Abuse & Incest National Network**
URL: www.rainn.org
Phone: (800) 656-HOPE, (202) 544-3064
Address: 2000 L Street NW, Suite 406, Washington, DC 20036
E-mail: info@rainn.org
Program: Operates the National Sexual Assault Hotline and Online
Hotline providing free, confidential information

**Self-Harmers' Hotline**
URL: www.selfinjury.com
Phone: (800) 442-HOPE, (800) DONTCUT

E-mail: info@selfinjury.com
Program: Help for self-injury through its confidential crisis hotline

## The Skin Cancer Foundation
URL: www.skincancer.org
Phone: (212) 725-5176
Address: 149 Madison Avenue, Suite 901, New York, NY 10016
E-mail: info@skincancer.org
Mission: To educate public and medical professionals about skin cancer prevention, early detection, and effective treatment
Program: Tour bus provides screening; Web site with information on all types of skin cancers; training; conferences; e-newsletter

# GLOSSARY

**abstinence**   the practice of not engaging in sexual relations or not drinking

**active immunization**   production of antibodies in response to the presence of antigens resulting in long-lasting **immunity**

**acute**   sudden onset or short term

**addiction**   a condition in which a person habitually gives in to a psychological, emotional, or physical need for a substance such as alcohol, tobacco, or drugs

**agoraphobia**   severe **anxiety** about being in open or public areas; literally means "a fear of the marketplace"

**Alateen**   a 12-step support program devoted to teenage family members and friends of alcoholics; the group uses the **Alcoholics Anonymous** model

**Alcoholics Anonymous (AA)**   the first and largest self-help group for alcoholics

**allergen**   a substance that triggers an allergy

**alveoli**   the final branches of the lung tree where oxygen and carbon dioxide are exchanged

**anaphylactic shock**   an often severe and sometimes fatal reaction affecting the respiratory system and causing raised patches of skin and intense itching in response to an **antigen**

**anorexia nervosa**   a medical and/or psychological condition in which a patient is unwilling to eat the minimum amount of food necessary to stay alive and healthy due to the mistaken idea that he or she is obese; sometimes associated with the abuse of alcohol

**antibiotics**   substances that destroy or slow the growth of **bacteria**

**antibodies**   produced by the body's **immune system** which bind to a specific foreign substance to fight **infection**

**antidepressant**   medication used to treat depression

**antigen**   foreign organism that can trigger an **immune response** from the body

**antihistamine**   medication that counteracts **histamine** in the body; used to treat allergic reactions and cold symptoms

**anti-inflammatory**   agent that reduces swelling, pain, redness, and heat associated with injury

**antioxidants**   substances that stop the oxidation of molecules that produces free radicals, which can harm cells

**anxiety**   when in response to real, versus imagined, situations, a normal reaction to stress that can help one deal with a tense circumstance, such as studying hard or focusing on something important

**anxiety disorder**   abnormal sense of fear, doubt about reality of the source of the fear, and self-doubt about coping with it

**arteriosclerosis**   narrowing of coronary arteries due to buildup of deposits in them

**bacteria**   single-celled organisms with no membranes around their genetic material; some are helpful, others cause disease

**bacterial pneumonia**   inflammation of the lungs caused by **bacteria**

**binge-eating disorder**   a mental condition in which a person periodically consumes huge amounts of food in a short period of time

**biopsy**   a procedure during which a needle is inserted into a suspicious area and the specimen sent to a laboratory for testing for the cells to see if abnormal cells exist in that area

**bipolar disorder**   a brain disorder that causes unusual shifts in a person's mood, energy, and ability to function; also known as manic-depressive illness

**body mass index (BMI)**   a scale that uses a person's height and weight to assess body fat in order to determine whether he or she is at a healthy weight or is underweight, overweight, or obese

**bulimia**   a medical and psychological condition in which the patient subjects his or her body to cycles of binge eating followed by vomiting or other extreme measures to get rid the excess food; often associated with alcohol abuse

**carcinogen**   substance or agent that causes cancer

**cardiovascular disease**   any illness involving the heart and blood vessels

**carrier**   transmitter of an infectious agent or a **gene**; the individual carrying the agent or gene has immunity to the disease or negative effect of the gene

**cell-mediated immunity**   condition in which various types of white blood cells fight **pathogens**

**chemotherapy**   the chemical treatment of disease, especially cancer

**chlamydia**   Sexually transmitted disease caused by **bacteria**

**cholera**   bacterial disease causing severe diarrhea

**cholesterol** a necessary fatlike substance made by the body and found naturally in certain foods such as meat and dairy products; high levels of cholesterol can lead to heart disease

**chromosomes** made of protein and DNA, threadlike structure in cells which carries genetic information

**chronic** long-lasting or repeated; used to describe any illness that is not easily cured

**cirrhosis** a **chronic** liver disease that occurs when the liver is scarred so that it cannot process and clean the blood as it normally does; often occurs as a consequence of alcohol abuse

**congenital** existing from birth

**contagious** communicable by contact

**computerized tomography (CT)** scanner that produces 3-D images of the inside of the body

**cornea** the clear front part of the eye covering the iris and pupil

**corticosteroids** **hormones** secreted by the adrenal cortex to regulate stress response, **immune response, inflammation,** and **metabolism**

**dehydration** abnormal loss of body fluids

**delirium tremens (DTs)** intense, terrifying hallucinations that can accompany withdrawal from alcohol or drugs, along with high fevers and extremely aggressive behavior

**dementia** progressive mental deterioration, including memory loss, confusion, reduction of the ability to handle everyday tasks, and variations in alertness

**depressant** a drug, including alcohol, tranquilizers, and inhalants, that lowers one's level of mental and physical activity, by quieting and depressing the central nervous system

**depression**   a mental condition characterized by feelings of extreme sadness or worthlessness, loss of interest in pleasurable activities, changes in sleep or appetite patterns, fatigue, and difficulty in concentrating

**detoxification**   a course of treatment, usually in a hospital or other facility, aimed at freeing people from drug or alcohol abuse and restoring their bodies to good health

**DNA (deoxyribonucleic acid)**   carrier of genetic material determining the inheritance of traits; contained in the **chromosomes** of all body cells except red blood cells

**dopamine**   brain chemical that helps transmit messages between brain cells

**Down syndrome**   disorder caused by a chromosomal problem that results in mental retardation, distinctive physical features, and usually health complications

**Ebola**   virus that causes infection that is passed between persons by direct contact with infected blood, body secretions, or organs

**enablers**   those around an addicted person who are manipulated by the addict into assisting the addict in continuing his or her habit

**enzyme**   protein that facilitates chemical reactions

**extrinsic attack**   a type of asthma attack triggered by outside influences such as allergies to pollen, dust, mold spores, or animal dander

**fetal alcohol syndrome**   a combination of birth defects caused by the mother's consumption of alcohol during pregnancy

**folate**   a water-soluble form of vitamin B9, found in high concentrations in spinach, lettuces, peas, beans, and asparagus

**fungi**   group of organisms that usually grow in moist conditions; some fungi can infect humans and cause disease

**gene**   biological unit that directs production of a particular protein and determines the presence or absence of a particular trait

**generalized anxiety disorder (GAD)**   a mental illness consisting of more severe worry and tension than most people experience

**gene swapping**   passing genetic material between two organisms, neither of which is an offspring; also called horizontal gene transfer

**gene therapy**   inserting of **genes** into cells in an effort to treat inherited disease or cancer

**genetics**   the DNA makeup of an organism

**hallucination**   a sight or sound of something that is not really there

**hemoglobin**   protein that moves oxygen from the lungs to the tissues and moves carbon dioxide (waste) from the tissues to the lungs

**hepatitis**   **inflammation** of the liver usually caused by a **virus**

**histamine**   chemicals released into bloodstream in response to allergic reactions, such as rashes, runny noses, and wheezing; causes blood vessels to open up, smooth muscles to constrict, and the stomach to produce acid

**hormone**   a chemical substance that some cells in the body release to help other cells work; for example, **insulin** is a hormone that helps the body use glucose as energy

**hyperactivity**   condition of excessive physical activity, which may be purposeful or aimless

**hyperglycemia**   abnormally high level of glucose in the bloodstream; inadequate **insulin** or the inability of insulin to carry glucose out of bloodstream into the body

**hypoglycemia**   a physical disorder in which blood glucose burns up too rapidly, and the body does not produce enough sugar

**immune response**   reaction when an **antigen** is recognized as a foreign invader and **antibodies** and lymphocytes capable of making it harmless are formed

**immune system**   the cells and organs in the body that fight disease and infection

**immunity**   resistance to disease that is achieved by the body's **immune system**

**immunotherapy**   treatment for or the prevention of disease by producing active or passive **immunity**

**incubation period**   time between initial exposure to **bacteria** and the development of the disease

**infection**   the growth of a parasitic organism within the body

**infectious**   capable of spreading to others

**inflammation**   response triggered by the **immune system** when white blood cells move to a wound or other area of infections; inflamed tissue is warm, red, and swollen

**insulin**   the **hormone** produced by the pancreas that helps convert glucose (sugar) in the body into energy

**insulin resistance**   situation in which cell receptors on the outside of cells do not allow usual access of **insulin** into cell interior; usually present before and during Type 2 diabetes

**interferon**   a drug that boosts the immune system's ability to fight cancer by binding to neighboring cells and stimulating those cells to produce antiviral proteins that prevent viruses from replicating in those cells

**intrinsic attack**   a type of asthma attack triggered by exercise, sports activities, extreme weather conditions, fatigue, or stress

**jaundice**   condition in which the skin yellows, caused by damage to the liver

**joints**  parts of the human body where two bones make contact; to allow for movement

**ketoacidosis**  an imbalanced body state in which the ketone proteins build up creating an acidic state in the Type 1 diabetic

**macula**  an oval-shaped spot in the center of the **retina** with a high concentration of cone cells, allowing for color vision and a high degree of visual sharpness

**magnetic resonance imaging (MRI)**  use of a combination of radio waves and a strong magnetic field to form an image of the inside of the body

**malignant**  tending to infiltrate and terminate fatally

**mania**  a distinct period of abnormally and persistently elevated, expansive, or irritable mood lasting at least one week

**metabolism**  the physical and chemical process in the body that breaks down substances in the body for generating and using energy; includes nutrition, digestion, absorption, elimination, respiration, circulation, and temperature regulation

**metastasis**  spread of cancer to other parts of the body

**microsurgery**  type of surgery performed with very small instruments while surgeons look at magnified images through a microscope

**muscular dystrophy**  heredity disorder characterized by degeneration of skeletal muscles

**mutation**  change in genetic material of a cell or organism that is inherited

**naturopathic**  an approach to healthcare that emphasizes natural remedies that do not rely on traditional medicine or surgery

**neurotransmitter**  a chemical that allows nerve cell to communicate with one another to maintain normal physical and psychological functioning

**norepinephrine**  a **hormone** and a **neurotransmitter**; as a hormone, secreted by the adrenal gland, it works alongside epinephrine (adrenaline) to give the body sudden energy in times of stress, known as the "fight or flight" response; as a neurotransmitter, it gives one a sense of emotional and physical fulfillment

**over-the-counter**  medication that can be purchased without a prescription

**pancreatitis**  inflammation or infection of the pancreas

**parasite**  organisms that live off of other organisms; they depend on the host organism for survival

**parasitic worm**  group of the largest **infectious** agents that includes roundworms, tapeworms, and hookworms

**passive immunization**  type of **immunity** acquired by transfer of **antibodies**

**pathogen**  agent of disease

**physical therapy**  physical and mechanical method of treating disease including stretching, exercise, massage, and water, light, heat, and electricity

**physiotherapy**  physical therapy

**plaque**  buildup of material that can block a coronary artery

**plasma**  fluid part of blood (as compared to the suspended portion)

**post-traumatic stress disorder (PTSD)**  a mental disorder that may result from experiencing or witnessing a life-threatening event such as sexual, physical, or emotional abuse, military combat, a natural disaster, a terrorist action, a serious accident, or a violent assault such as rape; symptoms include nightmares and flashbacks, difficulty sleeping, and feelings of detachment

**prediabetes**  condition of having the symptoms that will develop into a diagnosis of diabetes

**protists**   one-celled organisms, some of which are disease agents

**psychotherapy**   a course of treatment that includes the interaction between a therapist and a client to resolve symptoms of a mental disorder

**psychotropic drugs**   drugs that act in a particular way on the brain and affect the mind

**quarantine**   a restraint on the activities of a person to prevent the spread of disease, or the place in which those under quarantine are kept

**rehabilitation**   process of restoring to a former condition of health

**remission**   state of health after **chemotherapy,** radiation, and other medicines or therapies have destroyed all of the cancer cells

**reservoir hosts**   a person or animal in which an **infectious** agent, such as a **bacteria** or **virus,** multiples before transmission; the host suffers no ill effects

**respiratory**   of or relating to the circulation of air by breathing

**retina**   light-sensitive inner layer of the eye containing rod cells and cone cells, which transmit visual information to the optic nerve

**sedentary**   sitting or remaining inactive for long periods of time

**stem cell therapy**   treatment that involves replacing diseased cells with unspecialized cells able to develop into specialized cells; stem cells may have the ability to develop into limited types or any type of body cells

**steroid**   type of fatty chemical that includes **hormones** and bile; sometimes used to increase muscle mass and strength

**stimulant**   a drug, such as caffeine, nicotine, amphetamine, or cocaine, that tends to temporarily increase alertness, energy, and physical activity

**toxic shock syndrome** an uncommon bacterial infection that can affect anyone with a staph infection

**triglyceride** made from glycerol and three fatty acids, a molecule that is metabolized when the body needs a fatty acid energy source

**tumor** an abnormal tissue mass

**ultrasound** with a frequency of more than 20,000 hertz, sound waves that are used to diagnose and treat diseases; a two-dimensional image forms that helps examine and measure internal body structures

**vaccination** use of material to cause the **immune system** to develop resistance to **infection** by disease-causing organisms

**vaccine** killed or weakened disease-causing organism or materials that can be used to stimulate the **immune system** to develop resistance

**vector** a living thing or object which passes along a disease but is not itself affected by the disease

**virus** microscopic particles that can infect cells and reproduce inside the cells

# INDEX

Page numbers in **boldface** denote main entries.